MEDICINAL CHEMISTRY

Edited by **Janka Vašková**
and **Ladislav Vaško**

Medicinal Chemistry
http://dx.doi.org/10.5772/intechopen.76494
Edited by Janka Vašková and Ladislav Vaško

Contributors

Kimberly Suzanne George Parsons, Rebekah Wood, Rebecca Greenstein, Isabella Hildebrandt, Anab Fatima, Muhammad Jiyad Shaikh, Hina Zahid, Ishart Younus, Sheikh Abdul Khaliq, Farah Khalid, Shaymaa Kassab, Maria Dolors Pujol, Elisabet Batlle, Enric Lizano, Miquel Viñas, Xochitl Sofia Ramirez Gomez, Esmeralda Rodríguez-Miranda, Gabriel Herrera-Pérez, Rafael Vargas-Bernal, Sandra Neli Jimenez Garcia, Vicente Beltran Campos, Manon Mani Vellingiri, Parimala Gnana Soundari A, Tamilarasi S, Shui-Yuan Lu, Pinpin Lin, Chen-Yi Weng, Wei-Ren Tsai, Rinat Islamov, Alexander Ilin, Bahyitzhan Kerimzhanova, Janka Vašková, Ladislav Vaško

First published in London, United Kingdom, 2019 by IntechOpen
IntechOpen is the global imprint of INTECHOPEN LIMITED, registered in England and Wales, registration number: 11086078, The Shard, 25th floor, 32 London Bridge Street
London, SE19SG – United Kingdom
Printed in Croatia

British Library Cataloguing-in-Publication Data
A catalogue record for this book is available from the British Library

Additional hard copies can be obtained from orders@intechopen.com

Medicinal Chemistry, Edited by Janka Vašková and Ladislav Vaško
p. cm.
Print ISBN 978-1-78985-173-1
Online ISBN 978-1-78985-174-8

For EU product safety concerns:
IN TECH d.o.o., Prolaz Marije Krucifikse Kozulić 3, 51000 Rijeka, Croatia,
info@intechopen.com or visit our website at intechopen.com.

Meet the editors

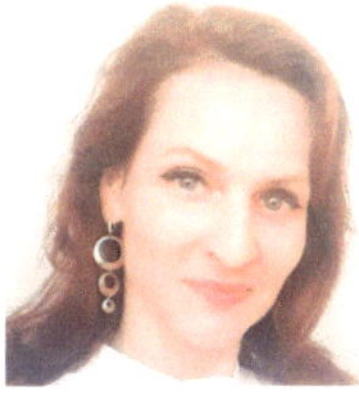

Associate Professor Dr. Janka Vašková has completed her PhD in Anthropology. She was appointed Associate Professor in Anthropology in 2016, and received the same scientific qualification level, senior researcher, in clinical biochemistry. She is working as a research scientist in the Department of Medical and Clinical Biochemistry, Faculty of Medicine at Pavol Jozef Šafarik University in Kosice. She is the author of three monographs/book chapters, four textbooks, and more than 280 original scientific and conference papers. Currently, she deals with the detection of pro- and antioxidant properties of natural and synthetic substances, their effect on the antioxidant status of the organism, as well as assessment of treatment success and patient prognosis by detecting the changes in selected antioxidant markers.

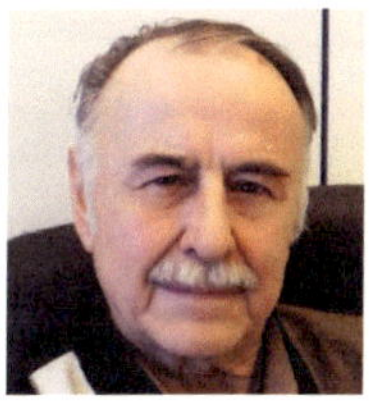

Ladislav Vaško, Associate Professor, DVM, PhD, has been working at the Clinic of Internal Diseases since graduation from the University of Veterinary Medicine in Košice. After doctoral studies he taught chemistry at the Department of Biochemistry and Toxicology. He was appointed Associate Professor in Biochemistry by the Ministry of Education of the Slovak Republic, and in 2006 habilitated to Associate Professor in Physiology and Morphology. Since 2008 he has been working at the Faculty of Medicine in Košice. He is the author of three monographs/book chapters, nine textbooks, and more than 420 scientific and conference papers. Currently, he deals with the effects of humic acids on organisms with simultaneous intake of toxic substances.

Contents

Preface

The area covered by this book undoubtedly includes a multidisciplinary approach. It combines and uses the wide range of methods and knowledge from a variety of disciplines in chemistry, pharmacology, and biology to synthesize new or extracted natural substances and their characterization, in terms of bioefficiency in different systems, pharmacokinetics, and pharmacodynamics. Importance is placed on revealing the interactions and effects on organisms. The process is long term, ranging from synthesis to potential testing of substances in animal studies, followed by monitoring effects on patients. The purpose is to define molecular targets of the highest efficacy of the prepared drugs, minimizing the undesirable effects. The content of this book is conceived with these intentions.

The introductory chapter deals with the use or monitoring of influence of production of reactive oxygen species by mitochondria after administration of newly prepared substances, which were devoted to this research by Prof. Perjési from Pécs (Hungary). Excessive and unmanageable production of reactive oxygen species leads to disruption of mitochondrial functions and induction of apoptosis. The chapter covers the monitoring of the efficacy of substances in biological systems in vitro. To illustrate the effects on cell substructures and energy production, the following chapters deal with the definition of cytotoxic effects of the isolated endophytic fungus *Aspergillus terrus* FC36AY1, as well as methylparaben, a substance used in cosmetics and UVB. Subsequently, the chapters deal with the development and effects of indomethacin-derived structures and derivatives derived from benzodiazepine and point to possible more pronounced and more targeted effects of these substances. Monitoring of the pharmacokinetics of known and used active substances at various concentrations and in combinations with other active substances as demonstrated in the chapter on clavulanic acid inactivating bacterial B-lactamase or novel iodine complex FS-1 as antituberculosis is another phase of research regarding organ distribution and the desired efficacy. Metabolism of ingested drugs and their bioavailability are mediated by cytochrome P450. The efficacy of its enzyme activity is directly related to the distribution and duration of action of these substances in organs. In this respect, it is necessary to know the effect of the activity of these enzymes on commonly ingested fruits and vegetables. The last part is dedicated to the authorized in vivo study of the endocrine disruption activity of three pesticides in rat embryos. This section also includes a chapter on the positive results of the proprioceptive neuromuscular facilitation method carried out on 15 football players on muscle stem cells and growth factor stimulation.

It is hoped that this book will be of benefit to all the readers for whom it is intended.

Janka Vašková, Assoc. Prof. Dr. PhD, and Ladislav Vaško, Assoc. Prof. DVM, PhD
Faculty of Medicine
Pavol Jozef Šafárik University
Košice, Slovak Republic

Introductory Chapter: Unregulated Mitochondrial Production of Reactive Oxygen Species in Testing the Biological Activity of Compounds

Janka Vašková and Ladislav Vaško

Additional information is available at the end of the chapter

http://dx.doi.org/10.5772/intechopen.82514

1. Introduction

Medicinal chemistry is an area that creates important links between the function of living organisms and the action of substances, whether natural or synthetic. This includes studies of structure–activity and dose–response associations in cell culture systems, in vitro and subsequent in vivo studies. The treatment of many diseases requires continuous invention, synthesis, characterization, and final testing of new designed compounds. Recently, there is also growing interest in better and more targeted use of the rich spectrum of effective natural substances extracted from plants. Each study thus contributes to the characterization of the effects of substances in order to achieve the least possible side effects in interactions and metabolism but significant expected ones. Also, part of such studies has been carried out at our workplace, which show the necessary and complementary role of identifying the effects and use of these substances. In this way, we introduce a shortened preview of unregulated endogenous production of reactive oxygen and nitrogen species in the biological activity of compounds in mitochondria.

2. Reactive oxygen species production in mitochondria

Mitochondria are two membrane organelles present in all cells that have a nucleus. They are the energy center of the cells. Their primary role is the production of ATP in oxidative phosphorylation, and the basis of the aerobic oxidation is the citric acid cycle interconnection representing the final metabolic pathway of oxidation of all major nutrients to the respiratory chain where oxidation of reduced coenzymes results in ATP formation. By the process of oxidative phosphorylation, the mitochondria have an irreplaceable function in the formation of metabolic energy in the form of ATP. The electrodes released in this process from reduced substrates are transferred to O_2 via the H^+ pumps of the respiratory chain. Pumps (complexes I–IV) form a H^+ gradient through the internal mitochondrial membrane, and the electrochemical energy of this gradient is then used to synthesize ATP complex V, ATP synthase [1]. Gradual reduction of O_2 occurs through several interstages when reactive oxygen species (ROS) are formed. One-electron reduction of O_2 to superoxide radical ($O_2^{\bullet}-$) is thermodynamically more advantageous, even for substances with relative oxidation ability, so in the mitochondria, a number of electron donors potentially allow this reaction [2]. However, only a small number of mitochondrial electron transporters with thermodynamic potential to reduce O_2 actually act. In most cases, small-molecule electron transporters such as NADH, NADPH, reduced coenzyme ($CoQH_2$), and reduced glutathione (GSH) do not react with O_2 but regenerate it. Instead, $O_2^{\bullet}-$ production takes place on the redox-active prosthetic groups of proteins or electron-binding proteins such as $CoQH_2$, which is a kinetic factor that allows or prevents the reduction of O_2 molecules and determines the production of $O_2^{\bullet}-$ in the mitochondria [3]. The mechanism of mitochondrial production and release of H_2O_2 and $O_2^{\bullet}-$ can be seen as described in more detail in [4]. Overall, in aerobic metabolism, the mitochondrial oxidative phosphorylation system balances the reduction of O_2 to H_2O in maximizing ATP synthesis with the simultaneous production of ROS only to the amount required for cell signaling [5].

The major part of the mitochondrial ROS production is formed as a by-product of the respiration on the inner side of the inner mitochondrial membrane. Complex IV (cytochrome c oxidase), a terminal component of the electron transport chain, receives four electrons from cytochrome c and reduces one molecule of O_2 to two H_2O. The intermediates remain partially reduced until they are completely reduced and are not secreted in measurable amounts [6]. Historically, the $O_2^{\bullet}-$ producing complex III was described as the first site of ROS production—in the Q-cycle [7]. Theoretically, the oxidation of succinate by succinate dehydrogenase (complex II, SDH) leads to significant $O_2^{\bullet}-$ formation—but so far it has not been measured. Thus, it is not entirely clear whether SDH produces in situ mitochondrial ROS. Nevertheless, the production of ROS complex II is a significant source in many tissues via the reverse electron transport mechanism. This particular phenomenon results from a high membrane potential that thermodynamically favors complex II as a donor for complex I., thanks to which succinate supports production of ROS in complex I. Thanks to which succinate supports production of ROS in complex I [6]. Complex I (NADH dehydrogenase) is the main entry of electrons into the respiratory chain. It is a significant source of ROS, namely, $O_2^{\bullet}-$ and H_2O_2, although it is very complicated to find out whether it is the major source of ROS in mitochondria in vivo. All evidence of significant ROS production was obtained in in vitro studies [8].

The mitochondria also contain other sources, outside the respiratory chain that highlight ROS production. On the outer mitochondrial membrane, there are cytochrome b5 reductase and monoamine oxidase. Cytochrome b5 reductase is present in all mammalian tissues and is capable of production $O_2^{\bullet}-$ at a very high rate of about 300 $mmol.min^{-1}.mg$ of $protein^{-1}$. Monoamine oxidases (MAO-A and MAO-B) are also present in all tissues of mammals.

They catalyze the oxidation of biogenic amines while releasing H_2O_2 [9]. On the outside of the internal mitochondrial membrane, the conversion of dihydroorotate to orotate catalyzes the de novo synthesis of uridine monophosphate dihydroorotate dehydrogenase. It is considered to be the source of $O_2^{\bullet}-$ and H_2O_2, although its ability to produce $O_2^{\bullet}-$ requires further study. Also, part of a glycerophosphate shuttle, the mitochondrial glycerol-3-phosphate dehydrogenase, is present in all cells but with uneven expression and mediating the formation of H_2O_2 [10]. In the mitochondrial matrix, there is localized aconitase catalyzing the conversion of citrate to isocitrate within the Krebs cycle. Enzyme contains a Fe-S cluster that can be oxidized by $O_2^{\bullet}-$ but also H_2O_2 leading to $^{\bullet}OH$ production [11]. The subunit of lipoamide dehydrogenase from the ketoglutarate dehydrogenase complex, located on the inner side of the membrane turned into the mitochondrial matrix, produces $O_2^{\bullet}-$ and H_2O_2. The subunit of the pyruvate dehydrogenase complex, dihydrolipoyl dehydrogenase, is also a significant source of ROS [12].

Mitochondria and ROS signaling control cell homeostasis by regulating processes of physiological cell death (apoptosis), including autophagy however also that of survival. Damage of mtDNA, protein carbonylation, or lipid peroxidation due to increased ROS production have been documented in many studies, and due to the localization and metabolic role of the organelles, they can lead to an energy disaster of the cell. Therefore, the production of ROS by mitochondria is considered crucial for cell survival or death. Many proteins that mediate apoptosis and autophagy directly affect ROS signaling by translocation into the mitochondria compartment and subsequent modulation of pro- or antioxidant enzymes [9].

3. Testing compounds

Synthetic and natural substances can affect the production of ROS; alter the redox state of the cell and, depending on the extent of the oxidative change; affect proliferation; or induce apoptosis. Chalcones are intermediate products of biosynthesis of a wide variety of plant polyphenols, flavonoids. Chalcones, as α, β-unsaturated carbonyl compounds have a wide range of substituents. The cycles are connected by three strongly electrophilic carbons, and the whole system creates a linear or almost planar structure [13]. They also contain a keto-ethylene group (–CO–CH=CH–). They have conjugated double bonds and a fully delocalized π-electron system on both benzene rings [14]. Structure–activity studies have shown that the cytotoxicity of chiral analogues is affected by the shape of the molecules [15, 16]. The multimodal pharmacodynamic, structural diversity of synthetic and natural chalcones and the constitutive elements that create optimal toxicity vary for each class of chalcones, and there are no generally valid rules of relationship between structure and activity [17]. Changes in the structure create a high degree of diversity which, as was shown, is useful for the development of new drugs with better efficacy, lower toxicity, and good pharmacological action. Thus, chalcones have become of interest not only in the academic but also in the industrial sphere and are used as intermediates for the preparation of compounds having therapeutic utility. They are currently used in the treatment of viral, cardiovascular diseases, parasitic infections, pain, inflammation, and gastric cancer, as well as additives and cosmetic ingredients [14].

Some natural but also synthetic chalcones have demonstrated cytotoxic activity against tumor cell cultures by inhibiting cell growth. However, they are also effective as anticancer and chemopreventive agents in vivo [18–20]. The amount of clinically useful antitumor drugs exhibits a genotoxic effect based on their affinity to amino groups of nucleic acid, but chalcones exhibit a pronounced affinity to thiols [15]. These reactions can alter intracellular redox (redox signaling) that can modulate processes such as DNA synthesis, enzyme activation, selective gene expression, and cell cycle regulation [21]. Many of the pharmacological potentials of chalcones are not used yet.

Summarizing the current knowledge of chalcone efficiency and their cyclic analogues ((*E*)-2-arylmethylene-1-indanone, (E)-2-arylmethylene-1-tetralone, and (*E*)-2-arylmethylene-benzosuberone) with several types of substituents, our studies were then primarily focused on monitoring their effects on mitochondria with respect to the production of ROS and the subsequent effects on selected antioxidant markers and ATP production. As the primary organ of xenobiotic metabolism in the body is the liver, studies with 4′-methyl-, methoxy- [16], 4′-hydroxy- [22], and 4′-dimethylamino-cyclic analogues of chalcones [23] were provided on mitochondria isolated from the rat liver. Analogues with methyl substituents showed rather a protective, antioxidant effect. Observed insufficiency in the antioxidant system and the level of reduced glutathione and associated enzymes such as glutathione peroxidase and glutathione reductase were significantly induced by the presence of benzosuberone in all types of substituents. They act as uncouplers of mitochondrial respiration, thus reducing ATP production. 4′-Hydroxy and 4′-dimethylamino analogues of chalcones exhibited similarly toxic effects as (*E*)-2-arylidene-1-indanones. Chalcones with substituents that increase the electron density of the B-ring, such as methoxy, butoxy, or dimethylamino groups, do not exhibit significant reactivity to reactive species [24].

The current level of knowledge makes it possible to use some of these biological properties of chalcone derivatives influenced by the nature of their substitution, such as the ability to inhibit 12-lipoxygenase and cyclooxygenases with 2′-hydroxychalcones, 4′-hydroxychalcones, and 2′,4′-dihydroxychalcones. Selective inhibitory effects on arachidonic-induced platelet aggregation predict them as antithrombotic or anti-inflammatory agents [25]. Under the low pH, the amino group, which are conditions normally found in tumors, is in protonated form increasing β-carbon electrophilicity in enone linkage, thereby increasing its reactivity as nucleophile acceptor in Michael additions [15], for example, thiol groups. Substantial antiproliferative activity was observed for chalcones with substituted amino groups [26]. All benzosuberone cyclic analogues at incubation with mitochondria caused a significant decrease in reduced glutathione (GSH) levels and simultaneous increase in glutathione peroxidase (GPx) activities. Lowering GSH levels most clearly defines the conditions of strong oxidative stress and leads to changes in the redox potential of the cell [27]. Although many antioxidant defense systems exist in the mitochondria, their maintenance is energy demanding. The first condition is a sufficient amount of ATP needed to synthesize low molecular weight antioxidants and molecules that provide uptake of ROS and ROS by-products. Benzosuberone as well as indanone analogues acted in mitochondria as phosphorylation deactivators, thereby reducing ATP production. GSH itself is able to reduce reactive oxygen and nitrogen species (RNOS); however, it is synthesized only in cytosol. Although it easily passes through the outer mitochondrial membrane via porin channels, it cannot pass through the inner mitochondrial membrane into the matrix as the anion. Here, the 2-oxoglutarate antiport is applied [28]. By importing GSH, mitochondria lose an important intermediate of the Krebs cycle, which must be replaced by anaplerotic reactions. It is important to note that in experiments, we have been working with isolated mitochondria where transfer of de novo synthesized glutathione was not possible. However, the energy intensity to maintain the redox status was not reduced. $O_2^{\cdot}-$ produced in the mitochondrial matrix, the membrane space, and the outer mitochondrial membrane reacts with other electron acceptors such as NO but primarily leads to the production of H_2O_2. The local antioxidant capacity of peroxidases then determines oxidative damage or H_2O_2-mediated signaling. The GPx catalytic mechanism requires cyclic oxidation/reduction of cysteine or selenocysteine residues at the catalytic center where GSH is used as a cofactor and GSSG is formed. Reactivation through glutathione reductase (GR) requires a reduction potential of NADPH, whose production also requires energy. The presence of glucose-6-phosphate dehydrogenase (and also isocitrate dehydrogenase), a source of NADPH formation in mitochondria, have been proven [29], but the enzyme is extremely sensitive to H_2O_2 levels, leading to its inhibition [29]. Affection of ATP production and changes in GSH levels are associated with the affection of apoptosis, cell division, and growth [30]. According to the decrease in mitochondrial membrane potential, they are able to incorporate into the membrane and induce apoptosis [31]. Conversely, the reduction of ROS production in the mitochondria by partial uncoupling of oxidative phosphorylation, such as observed with tetralone analogues, is a protective mechanism and also corresponds to the measured values of antioxidant parameters.

4. Conclusion

As a result of our observations, (E)-2-arylidene-1-tetralone shows antioxidant and (E)-2-arylidene-1-benzosuberone significant pro-oxidant and cytotoxic properties regardless of the character of the substituent. The findings have contributed to the targeted synthesis of derivatives that are expected to enhance the effect due to structural modification. The mentioned cyclic analogues of chalcones served as a structural substrate, with the aromatic ring B being replaced by a ferrocene. In previous studies on various different ferrocene derivatives, some have been shown to exhibit surprisingly high toxicity and antiproliferative activity [32–34]. Among the unique derivatives available for study, the antiproliferative effect of the (E)-3-(ferroceneethylene)-4-chromanone was the most effective [35]. The pronounced effect of cell viability and colony formation of cancer cells in dose-dependent manner has been shown by 1,1′-bis[(1-oxoindane-2-ylidene) methyl] ferrocene. The mechanism by which tested ferrocenyl compounds could demonstrate these remarkable properties is probably based on their activity with RNOS, which subsequently affected the antioxidant mechanisms of mitochondria. In general, the activity of the compounds with respect to $^{\cdot}OH$ and nitric oxide (NO) was very weak but, however, marked toward $O_2^{\cdot}-$ and the peroxynitrite anion (ONO_2-). The 1,1′-bis[(1-oxoindane-2-ylidene) methyl]ferrocene and 1,1′-bis[(1-oxotetralin-2-ylidene) methyl] ferrocene were involved in the significant production of $O_2^{\cdot}-$, leading to increased activities of superoxide dismutase; additionally, 1,1′-bis[(1-oxoindan-2-ylidene)methyl] ferrocene also exhibited the lowest inhibition of NO and ONO_2-. In addition to preserved concentrations of GSH, the mechanism of action, especially in this most effective derivative, is likely to be the modulation of mitochondrial activity through the induction of nitrosative stress.

The demonstration from our workplace suggests a long-term process of characterizing the effects of compounds, which contributes only a small amount to their complex knowledge. That is why authors have been invited to create the content of this book to bring their work and theoretical experiences in this area through their chapters.

Author details

Janka Vašková* and Ladislav Vaško

*Address all correspondence to: janka.vaskova@upjs.sk

Faculty of Medicine, Pavol Jozef Šafárik University in Košice, Košice, Slovak Republic

References

[1] Brookes PS, Yoon Y, Robotham JL, Andres MW, Sheu SS. Calcium, ATP, and ROS: A mitochondrial love-hate triangle. American Journal of Physiology - Cellular Physiology. 2004;**287**(4):C817-C833. DOI: 10.1152/ajpcell.00139.2004

[2] Andreyev AY, Kushnareva YE, Starkov AA. Mitochondrial metabolism of reactive oxygen species. Biochemistry (Moscow). 2005;**70**(2):200-214. http://protein.bio.msu.ru/biokhimiya/contents/v70/full/70020246.html

[3] Murphy MP. How mitochondria produce reactive oxygen species. The Biochemical Journal. 2009;**417**(Pt 1):1-13. DOI: 10.1042/BJ20081386

[4] Vašková J, Vaško L, Kron I. Oxidative processes and antioxidative metaloenzymes. Antioxidant Enzyme. 2012:19-58. DOI: 10.5772/50995. InTech, Croatia

[5] Brookes PS, Darley-Usmar VM. Hypothesis: The mitochondrial NO·signaling pathway, and the transduction of nitrosative to oxidative cell signals: An alternative function for cytochrome C oxidase. Free Radical Biology and Medicine. 2002;**32**(4):370-374. DOI: 10.1016/S0891-5849(01)00805-X

[6] Kowaltowski AJ, de Souza-Pinto NC, Caastilho RF, Vercesi AE. Mitochondria and reactive oxygen species. Free Radical Biology and Medicine. 2009;**47**(4):333-343. DOI: 10.1016/j.freeradbiomed.2009.05.004

[7] Dröse S, Brandt U. The mechanism of mitochondrial superoxide production by the cytochrome bc1 complex. The Journal of Biological Chemistry. 2008;**283**(31):21649-21654. DOI: 10.1074/jbc.M803236200

[8] Kushnareva Y, Murphy AN, Andreyev A. Complex 1-mediated reactive oxygen species generation: Modulation by cytochrome c and NAD(P)+ oxidation-reduction state. The Biochemical Journal. 2002;**368**(Pt 2):545-553. DOI: 10.1042/BJ20021121

[9] Marchi S, Giorgi C, Suski JM, Agnoletto C, Bononi A, Bonnora M, et al. Mitochondria-Ros crosstalk in the control of cell death and aging. Journal of Signal Transduction. 2012; **2012**(329635):1-17. DOI: 10.1155/2012/329635

[10] Mráček T, Pecinová A, Vrbacký M, Drahota Z, Houstek J. High efficiency of ROS production by glycerolphosphate dehydrogenase in mammalian mitochondria. Archives of Biochemistry and Biophysics. 2009;**481**(1):30-36. DOI: 10.1016/j.abb.2008.10.011

[11] Vásquez-Vivar J, Kalyanaraman B, Kennedy MC. Mitochondrial aconitase is a source of hydroxyl radical. An electron spin resonance investigation. Journal of Biological Chemistry. 2000;**275**(19):14064-14069. DOI: 10.1074/jbc.275.19.14064

[12] Starkov AA, Fiskum G, Chinopoulos C, Lorenzo BJ, Browne SE, Patel MS, et al. Mitochondrial alpha-ketoglutarate dehydrogenase complex generates reactive oxygen species. The Journal of Neuroscience. 2004;**24**(36):7779-7788. DOI: 10.1523/JNEUROSCI.1899-04.2004

[13] Cheng MS, Li RS, Kenyon G. A solid phase synthesis of chalcones by Claisen-Schmidt condensations. Chinese Chemical Letters. 2000;**11**(10):851-854

[14] Yerragunta V, Kumaraswamy T, Suman D, Anusha V, Patil P, Samhitha T. A review on chalcones and its importance. PharmaTutor. 2013;**1**(2):54-59

[15] Dimmock JR, Zello GA, Oloo EO, Quail JW, Kraatz H-B, Perjési P, et al. Correlations between cytotoxicity and various physicochemical parameters of some 2-arylidenebenzocyclanones determined by X-ray crystallography. Journal of Medicinal Chemistry. 2002;**45**(14):3103-3111. DOI: 10.1021/jm010559p

[16] Perjési P, Das U, De Clercq E, Balzarini J, Kawase M, Sakagami H, et al. Design, synthesis and antiproliferative activity of some 3-benzylidene-2,3-dihydro-1-benzopyran-4-ones which display selective toxicity for malignant cells. European Journal of Medicinal Chemistry. 2008;**43**(4):839-845. DOI: 10.1016/j.ejmech.2007.06.017

[17] Ni L, Meng CQ, Sikorski JA. Recent advances in therapeutic chalcones. Expert Opinion on Therapeutic Patents. 2004;**14**(2):1669-1691. DOI: 10.1517/13543776.14.12.1669

[18] Dimmock JR, Elias DW, Beazely MA, Kandepu NM. Bioactivities of chalcones. Current Medicinal Chemistry. 1999;**6**(12):1125-1149

[19] Middleton E Jr, Kandaswami C, Theoharides TC. The effect of plant flavonoids on mammalian cells: Implications for inflammation, heart disease, and cancer. Pharmacological Reviews. 2000;**52**(4):673-751

[20] Go ML, Wu X, Liu XL. Chalcones: An update on cytotoxic and chemopreventive properties. Current Medicinal Chemistry. 2005;**12**(4):483-499

[21] Powis G, Briehl M, Oblong J. Redox signaling and the controlof cell growth and death. Pharmacology & Therapeutics. 1995;**68**(1):149-173. DOI: 10.1016/0163-7258(95)02004-7

[22] Guzy J, Vaskova-Kubálková J, Rozmer Z, Fodor K, Mareková M, Poskrobová M, et al. Activation of oxidative stress response by hydroxyl substituted chalcones and cyclic chalcone analogues in mitochondria. FEBS Letters. 2010;**584**(3):567-570. DOI: 10.1016/j.febslet.2009.11.098

[23] Vašková J, Reisch R, Vaško L, Poškrobová M, Kron I, Guzy J, et al. Effect of selected dimethylaminochalcones on some mitochondrial activities. In Vitro Cellular & Developmental Biology. Animal. 2013;**49**(5):354-359. DOI: 10.1007/s11626-013-9600-x

[24] Patil CB, Mahajan SK, Katti SA. Chalcone: A versatile molecule. Journal of Pharmaceutical Sciences and Research. 2009;**1**(3):11-22. DOI: 10.1.1.180.3821

[25] Jantan I, Bukhari SN, Adekoya OA, Sylte I. Studies of synthetic chalcone derivatives as potential inhibitors of secretory phospholipase A2, cyclooxygenases, lipoxygenase and proinflammatory cytokines. Drug Design, Development and Therapy. 2014;**8**:1405-1418. DOI: 10.2147/DDDT.S67370

[26] Xia Y, Yang ZY, Xia P, Bastow KF, Nakanishi Y, Lee KH. Antitumor agents. Part 202: Novel 2′-amino chalcones: Design, synthesis and biological evaluation. Bioorganic & Medicinal Chemistry Letters. 2000;**10**(8):699-701. DOI: 10.1016/S0960-894X(00)00072-X

[27] Stone JR, Yang S. Hydrogen peroxide: A signaling messenger. Antioxidants & Redox Signaling. 2006;**8**(3-4):243-270. DOI: 10.1089/ars.2006.8.243

[28] Lash LH, Putt DA, Matherly LH. Protection of NRK-52E cells, a rat renal proximal tubular cell line, from chemical-induced apoptosis by overexpression of a mitochondrial glutathione transporter. The Journal of Pharmacology and Experimental Therapeutics. 2002;**303**(2):476-486. DOI: 10.1124/jpet.102.040220

[29] Mailloux RJ, Harper ME. Glucose regulates enzymatic sources of mitochondrial NADPH in skeletal muscle cells; a novel role for glucose-6-phosphate dehydrogenase. The FASEB Journal. 2010;**24**(7):2495-2506. DOI: 10.1096/fj.09-151803

[30] Lash LH. Mitochondrial glutathione transport: Physiological, pathological and toxicological implications. Chemico-Biological Interactions. 2006;**163**(1-2):54-67. DOI: 10.1016/j.cbi.2006.03.001

[31] Kubálková J, Tomečková V, Perjési P, Guzy J. Assessment of the effect of cyclic chalcone analogues on mitochondrial membrane and DNA. Central European Journal of Biology. 2009;**4**(1):90-96. DOI: 10.2478%2Fs11535-008-0057-y

[32] Gasser G, Ott I, Metzler-Nolte N. Organometallic anticancer compounds. Journal of Medicinal Chemistry. 2011;**54**(1):3-25. DOI: 10.1021/jm100020w

[33] Goitia H, Nieto Y, Villacampa MD, Kasper C, Laguna A, Gimeno MC. Antitumoral gold and silver complexes with ferrocenylamide phosphines. Organometallics. 2013;**32**(20):6069-6078. DOI: 10.1021/om400633z

[34] Jaouen G, Top S, Vessières A, Leclercq G, MJ MG. The first organometallic selective estrogen receptor modulators (SERMs) and their relevance to breast cancer. Current Medicinal Chemistry. 2004;**11**(18):2505-2517. DOI: 10.2174/0929867043364487

[35] Vašková J, Žatko D, Vaško L, Perjési P, Poráčová J, Mojžišová G. Some ferrocenyl chalcones as useful candidates for cancer treatment. In Vitro Cellular & Developmental Biology. Animal. 2015;**51**(9):964-974. DOI: 10.1007/s11626-015-9919-6

Section 1

Effects on Biological Systems: In Vitro Testing

Chapter 2

Determination of *In Vitro* Cytotoxicity and Anti-Angiogenesis for a Bioactive Compound from *Aspergillus terreus* FC36AY1 Isolated from *Aegle marmelos* around Western Ghats, India

Vellingiri Manon Mani,
Arockiam Jeyasundar Parimala Gnana Soundari and
Selvam Tamilarasi

Additional information is available at the end of the chapter

http://dx.doi.org/10.5772/intechopen.81046

Abstract

The biotechnological research mainly emphasis its investigation on searching new natural drugs at economical to human welfare. With this view in mind, this research has focused to develop a prospective bioactive compound isolating from an efficient endophytic fungus isolated from potential medicinal tree *Aegle marmelos*. The endophytic fungus was isolated from the medicinal tree and identified as *Aspergillus terreus* FC36AY1. This fungus produced maximum of crude metabolites and this was produced in Sabouraud's Dextrose Broth. The produced metabolites were extracted using acetone as a sole solvent and it was taken for the assessment of antimicrobial and antioxidant analysis. The crude metabolites exhibited maximum activity at least concentration and further the crude extract were taken for purification processes through chromatographic techniques. Through purification, five different fractions were eluted and those five different fractions were also assessed for antimicrobial and antioxidant analysis. From these analysis results, TA4 was found to be efficient fraction and it was characterized through FT-IR, GC-MS and UV-VIS analysis. The compound was taken for cytotoxicity determination in HT-29 cancer cells and anti-angiogenesis analysis was assessed through HET-CAM testing. The bio-activities study revealed that the compound TA4 has the ability to target the cancer cells in an efficient manner.

Keywords: *Aspergillus* sp., cytotoxicity, metabolites, HPLC

1. Introduction

There are numerous natural pigments in the world. They are collected from the sources such as plants, animals and microorganisms. The uses of natural pigments are increasing worldwide. The natural pigments have several affecting factors like temperature, pH, availability and cost. The natural pigments do not cause any serious health effects but it may cause some side effects only for the hypersensitivity persons. The natural pigments are also called as secondary metabolites in which the plants and microbes will produce in enormous by the metabolic production. Each living organism undergoes several pathways for the production of useful secondary metabolites. In this way the best and economical source is microbial metabolites and they have been extensively used in pharmaceutical and medicinal fields to treat various disorders and diseases. With this focus in mind, this research has been focused on the purification of secondary metabolites from an endophytic fungus which would be isolated from an efficient medicinal tree from biodiversified place.

Microbial pigment production is now one of the emerging fields of research to demonstrate its potential for various industrial applications. Among the molecules produced by microorganisms are carotenoids, melanins, flavins, quinines and more specifically monascins, violacein or indigo. Industries are now able to produce some microbial pigments for applications in food, cosmetics and textiles. Naturally, pigment producing microorganisms like fungi, yeast and bacteria are quite common [1]. The pigments producing microorganisms will produce the antibiotic and inhibit the disease causing pathogens. Antibiotics eliminate or prevent the growth and can therefore cure disease caused by bacterial infection. They cannot however treat viral infection such as common cold or nonbacterial inflammation. Among the microbial pigments the fungi placed a promising rank for its largest and efficient production of potential metabolites which could be applicable in different medicinal and pharmaceutical industries. To which, endophytic fungi explored an evidence in the production of medically used metabolites mainly from medicinal plants. An endophyte is an endosymbiont that lives within a plant for at least part of its life cycle without causing apparent disease [2]. Endophytes are ubiquitous and have been found in all species of plants however, most of the endophyte/plant relationships are not well understood [3]. Endophytes are also known to occur within lichens [4] and algae [5]. Many economically important grasses (e.g., *Festuca* sp. and *Lolium* sp.) carry fungal endophytes in genus *Epichloë*, some of which may enhance host growth [6], nutrient acquisition and may improve the plant's ability to tolerate abiotic stresses, such as drought, and enhance resistance to insects, plant pathogens and mammalian herbivores. Nowadays the studies have focused on endophytic fungi isolated from medicinal tree. From ancient time onwards the medicines have been prepared from trees and plants in order to prevent/or cure the diseases. In this regard the current research has been focused on developing the medicine or drugs from the endophytic fungi residing in potential medicinal plants/or trees. These drugs are nothing but the metabolites produced from the metabolic pathways by the organisms. As the endophytes (i) mimics the metabolism of the host plant, (ii) easy for industrial means and (iii) improvement in activity compared to host plant. The drug derived from endophytes explores the nature of the drugs derived from the medicinal plants and/or trees. The research will be discussed on the bioactive secondary metabolites produced by endophytic fungi through different production, and their usage in different medicinal fields as anti-angiogenic product.

2. Materials and methods

2.1. Isolation and identification of endophytic fungi

The potential endophytic fungus was isolated from a prospective medicinal plant *Aegle marmelos* from Western Ghats (Nilgiris cluster), Coimbatore. This fungus was found to exhibit highest antagonistic activity when compared to other 37 different endophytic fungi from the medicinal plant. Further the potential fungus was named as FC36AY1 and identified to be *Aspergillus terreus* FC36AY1 with the NCBI accession number KY807648. The FC36AY1 was taken for the production of metabolites in Sabouraud's Dextrose Broth (SDB) medium for 17 days of incubation at stationary phase in normal cycle. The pigmented crude metabolites extract was extracted using acetone as sole solvent and it was concentrated for further use. The crude metabolites extract was assessed for biological determination such as antimicrobial and antioxidant analysis [7]. The fungus FC36AY1 manifested maximum activity at least concentration so this was taken for further purification process. The mass production of pigmented secondary metabolites was carried out in SDB medium and the yield was calculated according to Mani et al. [7]. The crude extract was taken for purification process to elute the bioactive secondary metabolite through chromatographic techniques.

2.2. Partial purification of the bioactive secondary metabolite

2.2.1. TLC

The crude extract was subjected to TLC (thin layer chromatography) [8]. About 5 μL of the crude extract was applied 1 cm above from the lower edge of the thin layer chromatography slides and dried. It was immersed to a depth of 1 cm in the solvents. The different solvent system tested for movement of the pigment was chloroform:methanol and petroleum ether:ethyl acetate. The best solvent system for the separation of the components in the crude extract was taken. The solvent front was marked and R_f value was calculated.

2.2.2. High performance liquid chromatography (HPLC)

The active fraction was further purified through preparative high performance liquid chromatography (HPLC) (Shimadzu-1100 series), manual injector with quaternary pump, photodiode array detector equipped with C_{18} column (4.6 × 250 mm) with 5 μL of pore size with the flow rate of 1 mL/min and mobile phase of acetonitrile:H_2O (80:20) at 427 nm.

2.3. Antioxidant activity

The purified fractions were taken for antioxidant analysis for determining the prospective secondary metabolite.

2.3.1. DPPH radical scavenging assay

The antioxidants present in fungal crude metabolites were aliquot into different concentrations (20–100 μg) to determine extract's ability to scavenge of 2,2-diphenyl-1-picrylhydrazyl

(DPPH) radicals using the method of Mani et al. [7] in triplicates. DPPH solution (1 mM DPPH radical solution in 95% ethanol) was added to the crude metabolites extracts and made upto 1 mL, vortexed well, and then incubated for 30 minutes in dark hood at room temperature. After incubation, the samples were poured into microfuge tubes and centrifuged for 5 min at 13,500 rpm at RT. The absorbance of each sample at $\lambda = 517$ nm was measured and 1 mL of 95% EtOH/MeOH was used as a control, and DPPH were used as reference compounds. The antioxidant activity is given as percent (%) DPPH scavenging assay was calculated using the formula: [(control absorbance − extract absorbance)/(control absorbance) × 100]. The fungi exhibiting the maximum antioxidant activity at minimum concentration and antagonistic profile were taken for further identification studies.

2.3.2. *Reducing power assay*

Total reducing power was determined as described by Oyaizu [9] in triplicates [7]. 1 mL of sample solution at different concentrations (20–100 μg) was mixed with 2.5 mL of phosphate buffer (0.2 mol/L, pH 6.6) and 2.5 mL of 1% potassium ferricyanide. The mixture was incubated at 50°C for 20 min, 2.5 mL of 10% trichloroacetic acid (TCA) was added to the mixture and centrifuged at 3000 × *g* for 10 min. The supernatant (5 mL) was mixed with 1 mL of ferric chloride (0.1%), and the absorbance was measured at 700 nm in a spectrophotometer. Increased absorbance of the reaction mixture indicated increased reducing power.

2.3.3. *Metal chelating activity*

The metal chelating activity was analyzed by the method of Dinis et al. [10] with slight modification in triplicates [7]. The reaction was performed in HEPES buffer (20 mM) at pH 7.2. Various concentrations (20–100 μg) of samples were mixed with a solution of 12.5 μM ferrous sulfate solution. Addition of 75 μM ferrozine was to initiate the reaction and the mixture was shaken vigorously and incubated for 20 min at room temperature. After incubation the absorbance was measured at 562 nm. Ascorbic acid was used as the reference compound and the percentage chelating capacity was calculated as; % chelating activity = $[(A_0 - A_1)/A_0] \times 100$ where, A_0 = absorbance of the blank; A_1 = absorbance of the sample.

2.3.4. *Superoxide anion radical scavenging assay*

Measurement of the superoxide anion radical scavenging capacity of the eluted fractions were essential according to the method described by Liu et al. [11] using a minor modification. The principle of this method is that superoxide radicals are generated in phenazine methosulfate (PMS)-nicotinamide adenine dinucleotide (NADH) systems by oxidation of NADH and reduction of nitroblue tetrazolium (NBT). In this experiment, the superoxide radicals were generated with 3.0 mL of Tris-HCl buffer (16 mM, pH 8.0) containing 1.0 mL of NBT (50 μM) solution, 1.0 mL NADH (78 μM) solution and samples of the compound MM4 (20–100 μg/mL) in methanol. The reaction was initiated by adding 1.0 mL of phenazine methosulfate (PMS) solution (10 μM) to the mixture. The absorbance at 560 nm was measured against a blank. Ascorbic acid was used as a standard. The scavenging activity was calculated by: [(Abs control − Abs sample)/Abs control] × 100.

2.3.5. *Hydroxyl radical scavenging assay*

The scavenging activity for hydroxyl radicals recommended by Yu et al. [12] was followed with minor changes using the fractions. Reaction mixture contained 0.6 mL of 1.0 mM Deoxy ribose, 0.4 mL of 0.2 mM phenyl hydrazine, 0.6 mL of 10 mM phosphate buffer (pH 7.4). It was incubated for 1 h at room temperature. Then 1 mL of 2–8% TCA, 1 mL of 1% TBA and 0.4 mL of compound (at different concentrations) were added and kept in water bath for 20 min. The absorbance of the mixture at 532 nm was measured with a spectrophotometer. From the readings, the hydroxyl radical scavenging activity was calculated as: [(Abs control − Abs sample)/Abs control] × 100.

2.3.6. *Chemical characterization of bioactive secondary metabolite*

The bioactive purified fraction which evinced maximum antioxidant activity at least concentration was dissolved in acetone and it was taken for UV-analysis using UV-Vis scanning spectroscopy for the detection of single peak. Scanning was performed between 200 and 800 nm wavelength. Later the fraction was subjected to structural elucidation of the compound. 1 mg of purified fraction was dried and analyzed for Infrared (IR) spectra using FTIR spectroscopy. The important IR bands of symmetric and asymmetric stretching and stretching frequencies were studied to determine the presence of functional groups.

The gas chromatography-mass spectrometry was done by advanced equipment (Thermo GC—Trace ultra VER: 5.0, Thermo MS DSQ II). The column used in this experiment was DB 5-MS capillary standard non-polar column with the dimension of 30 mts, ID-0.25 mm and the film was 0.25 μm. The carrier gas used was helium, with the flow rate at 1.0 mL/min and the temperature was as oven temperature 70°C which was raised to 260°C at 6°C/min. The sample of 1 μL which was purified from HPLC analysis was taken and injected for the experiment.

2.4. *In vitro* studies

2.4.1. *MTT assay*

The cytotoxic effect of the bioactive compound was studied using cancer cell lines. The HT-29 cell line was obtained from National Centre for Cell Sciences, Pune (NCCS). The cells were maintained in Minimal Essential Medium supplemented with 10% FBS, penicillin (100 U/mL), and streptomycin (100 μg/mL) in a humidified atmosphere of 50 μg/mL CO_2 at 37°C. Cells (1×10^5/well) were plated in 24-well plates and incubated in 37°C with 5% CO_2 condition. After the cell reaches the confluence, the various concentrations of the samples were added and incubated for 24 h. After incubation, the sample was removed from the well and washed with phosphate-buffered saline (pH 7.4) or MEM without serum. 100 μL/well (5 mg/mL) of 0.5% 3-(4,5-dimethyl-2-thiazolyl)-2,5-diphenyl-tetrazolium bromide (MTT) were added and incubated for 4 h. After incubation, 1 mL of DMSO was added in all the wells. The absorbance at 570 nm was measured with UV-Vis Spectrophotometer using DMSO as the blank. Measurements were performed and the concentration required to inhibit 50% of cells (IC_{50}) was determined graphically. The % cell viability was calculated using the following formula 1:

$$\%\text{cell viability} = \left(A_{570} \text{ of treated cells}/A_{570} \text{ of control cells} \times 100\right) \quad (1)$$

Graphs were plotted using the % of cell viability as Y-axis and concentration of the sample in X-axis. Cell control and sample control was included in each assay to compare the full cell viability in cytotoxicity assessments.

2.5. Determination of HET-CAM test [Hen's egg test on the chorio-allantoic membrane (HET-CAM) of chick eggs]

In order to understand the inflammatory tissue reactions of metabolite coated materials on the live tissues, the materials were placed on the surface of Chorio-Allantoic membrane (CAM) of embryonated chick eggs. The inflammatory response on CAM was evaluated by direct evaluation method. Freshly laid fertile eggs were collected from the chicken farm and incubated at 36–37°C for 8 days before implanting (implantation day: 9th day) the sample materials such as compound TA4, acetone, positive and negative solutions. During the incubation time, the eggs were turned twice daily. On the day of implantation (9th day after laid), the eggs were candled to determine the position of the air sac and the embryo. A square, with sides approximately 18–20 mm, was marked on the shell where the chorio-allantoic membrane was best developed. Using a dental drill fitted with a straight hand-piece the sides of the marked square were drilled. In one corner of this large triangle a second smaller square was drilled, with sides of approximately 5 mm. A small slit was drilled in the shell over the air sac.

2.5.1. Application of test sample, solvent, positive and negative control on CAM

Aseptic technique was used for the implantation of the test sample on biomaterial as filter paper discs. For dropping the material onto chorio-allantoic membrane the egg was mounted on a stand, with the drilled area of shell uppermost; a straight Hagedorn's needle was gently inserted under one corner of the smaller square of shell and this square was raised and removed. The shell and shell membrane circumscribed by the larger square were then removed, and the sterile pre-measured size of sample was inserted and carefully lowered on to the exposed membrane. In order to implement the implanted sample TA4, 0.3 mL of the substance (positive and negative control) was applied to the surface of the CAM on separate eggs. 0.1 N NaOH was added on the CAM of separate egg as a positive control and 0.9% NaCl was used as an appropriate negative control. After a 20-s exposure period, the CAM is rinsed with 5 mL of water.

2.5.2. Direct evaluation of CAM time for development of observed endpoints after exposure to the test substance

A procedure used to evaluate the time for development of endpoints after exposure to the test substance was to continually observe the CAM during the 5-min observation period and record (typically in seconds) the time at which each of the endpoints developed. Therefore, two separate time values (after 2 and 18 h of incubation) were obtained and recorded for each egg (one time value for each endpoint).

3. Results

3.1. Purification of secondary metabolite

3.1.1. Thin layer chromatography

The concentrated crude metabolite extract was subjected to thin layer chroamtography and the best solvent system which separated maximum compounds as band was chloroform:me thanol:toluene:acetic acid and at 95% about five visible bands got separated (**Figure 1a**)—R_f value was calculated for obtained peaks and tabulated (**Table 1**).

3.1.2. High performance liquid chromatography (HPLC)

The crude extract was forced for preparative HPLC analysis about 6 different peaks were obtained at 427 nm (**Figure 1b**) and this range corresponds to the result of UV spectrum analysis. The eluted fractions from HPLC analysis were assessed for antimicrobial profile. Among the five fractions (TA1–TA5), fraction 4 (TA4) was found to contain highest antimicrobial profile on comparing to other fractions (**Table 2**). The fraction 4 explored highest activity against *C. albicans, K. pneumoniae, E. coli, S. epidermidis* and *S. typhi.* From these results it is evident that this particular fraction was able to control the growth of gastro intestinal and skin pathogens.

3.2. Determination of antioxidant properties

3.2.1. DPPH radical scavenging activity

The bioactive compound of the present study showed a concentration dependent antiradical activity by inhibiting DPPH radical (**Figure 2a**). The decrease in absorbance of the DPPH radical

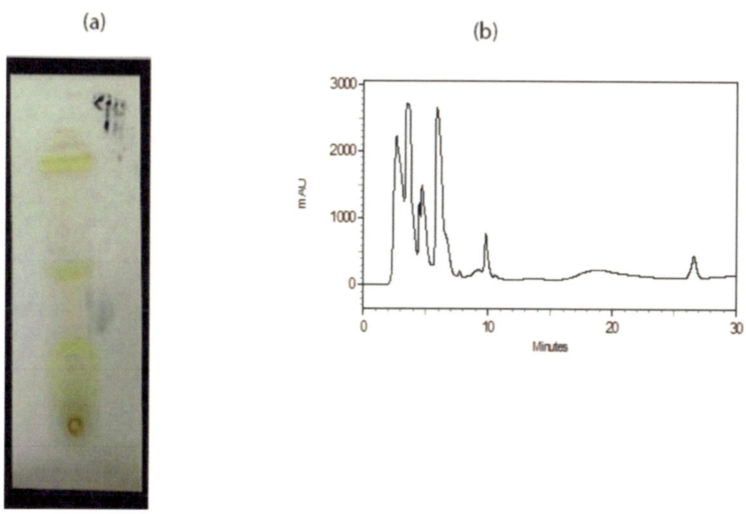

Figure 1. (a) TLC of crude extract and (b) chromatogram showing different peaks in *Aspergillus* sp. extract.

S. no.	Bands	R_f value (%)
1	I	0.046
2	II	1.125
3	III	1.184
4	IV	1.25
5	V	1.8
6	VI	1.956
7	VII	3.461
8	VIII	9.000

Table 1. R_f value of TLC for crude extract.

S. no.	Pathogens	Zone of inhibition (in cm)				
		TA1	TA2	TA3	TA4	TA5
1	*Staphylococcus aureus*	0.5	0	1.2	1.2	1.2
2	*Klebsiella pnuemoniae*	0	0	0.9	1.4	0.9
3	*Staphylococcus epidermis*	0.9	0	0.8	1.6	0
4	*Pseudomonas aeruginosa*	1.1	0	1.2	1.1	0
5	*Enterococcus faecalis*	1.2	0	2.1	2.1	0
6	*Bacillus subtilis*	1	0	0	2.3	1.3
7	*E. coli*	0	0	0	1.0	1.2
8	*Proteus mirabilis*	0	0	1.1	0.9	0.9
9	*Shigella sp*	0	0	0.9	0	0.7
10	*Salmonella*	0	0	0	0	0.8
11	*Candida albicans*	0	0	0	2.1	0.9
12	*Aspergillus terreus*	2.1	0	0	2.3	0

<0.5 cm: no inhibition activity.

Table 2. Antimicrobial activity for eluted fractions.

caused by antioxidant was due to the scavenging of the radical by hydrogen donation. It is visually noticeable as a color change from purple to yellow. Also, a lower value of IC_{50} (concentration at which the 50% scavenging activity is obtained) indicates a higher antioxidant activity at lower concentration. The IC_{50} concentration of purified fraction was found to 56 μg/mL.

3.2.2. Reductive power ability

The reducing ability of a bioactive compound generally depends on the presence of reductones, which exert the antioxidant activity by breaking the free radical chain by donating a

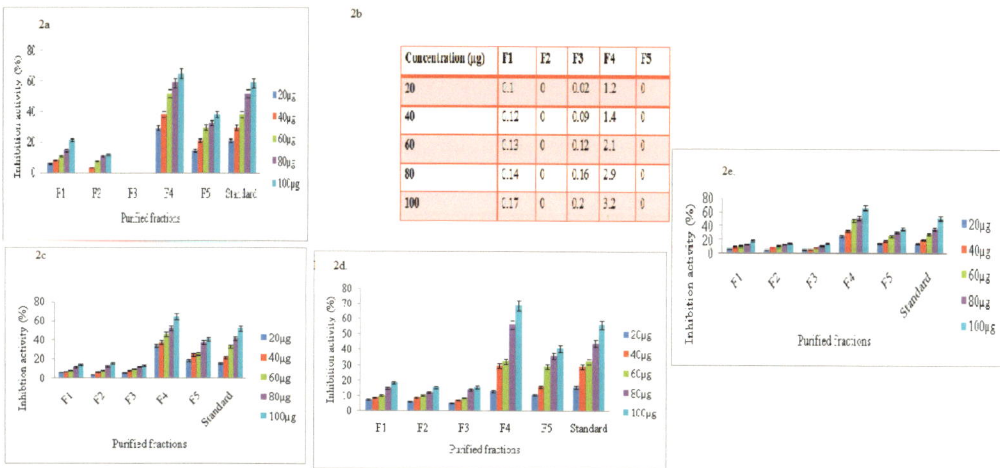

Concentration (μg)	F1	F2	F3	F4	F5
20	0.1	0	0.02	1.2	0
40	0.12	0	0.09	1.4	0
60	0.13	0	0.12	2.1	0
80	0.14	0	0.16	2.9	0
100	0.17	0	0.2	3.2	0

Figure 2. (a) DPPH radical scavenging activity, (b) reductive power ability of purified fraction, (c) superoxide radical scavenging activity, (d) hydroxyl radical scavenging activity, and (e) metal chelating activity.

hydrogen atom. In this study, the reductive ability of the compound TA4 had a maximum reductive power and this was observed by increasing OD units (**Figure 2b**). This confirmed the increasing reducing power through increasing OD units. When compared to the standard ascorbic acid, TA4 exerted a similar activity. This activity was concurrent with the investigation of ***Liu et al. (2007) with the same concentration of 20–100 μg/mL.

3.2.3. *Superoxide radical scavenging activity*

The superoxide radicals are generated by PMS and it was assessed using NBT. **Figure 2c** explains that the bioactive compound has a maximum scavenging mechanism at minimum concentration. The 50% of inhibition concentration value was found to be 24 μg/mL. The IC_{50} concentration of purified fraction was found to 68 μg/mL.

3.2.4. *Hydroxyl radical scavenging activity*

Hydroxyl radical scavenging assay showed the ability of the bioactive compound and standard ascorbic acid in inhibiting hydroxyl radical mediated deoxyribose degradation in a Fe^{3+} EDTA ascorbic acid and H_2O_2 reaction mixture (**Figure 2d**). The IC_{50} value of the compound was found distinctly increased with increased concentration when compared to the standard. Hydroxyl radicals are the major active oxygen species causing enormous biological damage by lipid peroxidation in cells. The IC_{50} concentration of purified fraction was found to 75 μg/mL.

3.2.5. *Metal chelating activity*

The rate of color reduction was measured which was used in the estimation of chelating activity of the coexisting chelator. In the current analysis, the absorbance of Fe^{2+} ferrozine complex was decreased in a dose dependent manner which can be meant in other way as the activity increased with the increasing concentration from 20 to 100 μg/mL and the IC_{50} concentration of purified fraction was found to 70 μg/mL (**Figure 2e**).

3.3. Chemical characterization of the secondary metabolite

UV-Visible spectrum of the purified pink colored compound was recorded using acetone solution in the range of 200–700 nm showed a single peak for the purified fraction (**Figure 3a**). The spectral measurement showed that the compound had registered its absorption band in the region 427 nm. The peak in the wavelength of 427 nm showed that this is the active fraction. IR spectrum has proven to be the most effective way to give the information about the functional groups present in the compound.

Figure 3b depicted the FT-IR report for the purified fraction. In that, the stretching frequencies of the IR spectrum recorded the highest peak at 1711.92 which correspond to C—O (carbonyl/ketone) stretching. The region 1360.41 denotes the region —C—H (sp^3 configuration and alkane group) and the region 1221.06 records CN stretching (aromatic primary amine group or phenolic group). The region 1426.80 and 1093.19 denotes —C—H (sp^3 configuration with vinyl C—H) and C—O (alcohol group) respectively. The frequencies from 3600 to 3200 cm^{-1} denoted the alcohol group present in the compound and in the same way the frequencies recorded from 3000 to 2850 cm^{-1} denoted the alkane stretching.

3.3.1. GC-MS analysis

The gas chromatography-mass spectrometry (GC-MS) was analyzed for purified fraction of TA4. The chromatogram was obtained with 4 major peaks in TA4 (**Figure 3c** and **d**). Finally from the results of UV-spectra, FT-IR, GC-MS, analysis we conclude the compound of TA4 was found to be octadecenoic acid 4-hydroxy methyl ester C19H38O3.

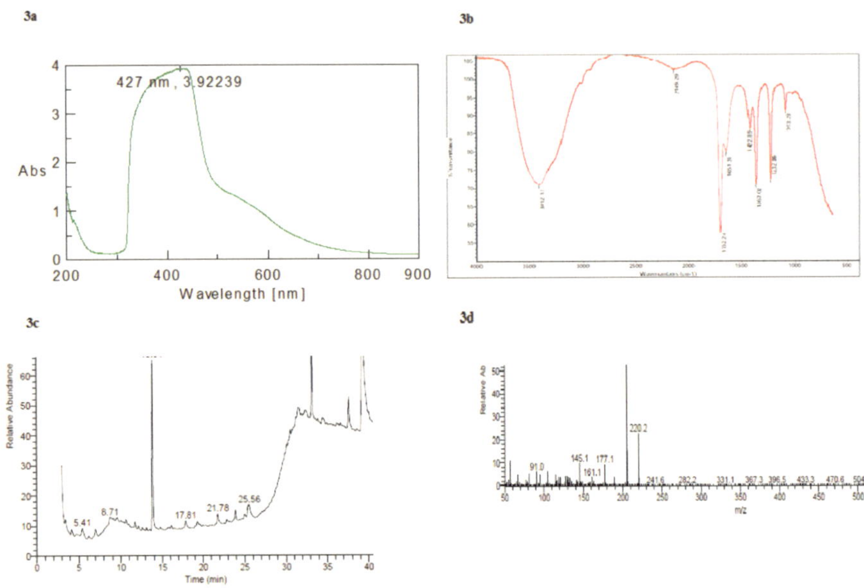

Figure 3. (a) UV-VS of TA4, (b) FT-IR spectra for TA4, (c) GC-MS of TA4, and (d) GC-MS RA peak of TA4.

3.4. *In vitro* studies

3.4.1. MTT assay

The present investigation has been carried out for a potential bioactive compound TA4. The studies have been performed on HT-29 colon cancer cell lines with the control of triton X 100 (**Table 3** and **Figure 4**). This result was similar to the investigation of Yuvaraj et al. [13] reported the IC_{50} at nearest concentration. The present study has showed that *A. terrus* FC36AY1 acetonic fractions could extensively inhibited cell proliferation architecture in dose dependent manner. This report demonstrating the *in vitro* anticancer activity of the TA4 from methanolic extract of *A. terrus* FC36AY1 providing a scientific basis for its effects on human health which is similar to Yuvaraj et al. [13], TA4 was found to be inhibited maximum number of cells. So TA4 was taken for further studies.

Sample concentration (μg/mL)	Average OD at 540 nm	Percentage viability
Control	0.3855	
6.25	0.3044	78.96239
12.5	0.2941	76.29053
25	0.2427	62.9572
50	0.2077	53.87808
100	0.1545	40.07782

Table 3. MTT assay.

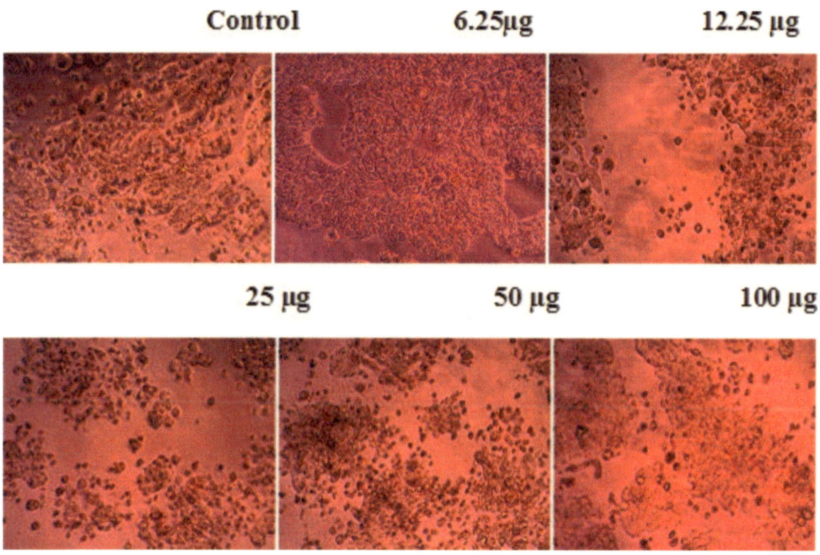

Figure 4. MTT analysis of TA4.

Sample	For 2 h		For 18 h	
	No. of vessels in untreated CAM	No. of vessels in treated CAM	No. of vessels in untreated CAM	No. of vessels in treated CAM
Negative control—acetone	18	10	18	05
Sample—1–200 μL	12	10	12	08
Sample—1–400 μL	10	05	13	03
Positive control—NaOH	11	11	11	11

Table 4. Anti-angiogenesis effect of TA4 in HET-CAM test.

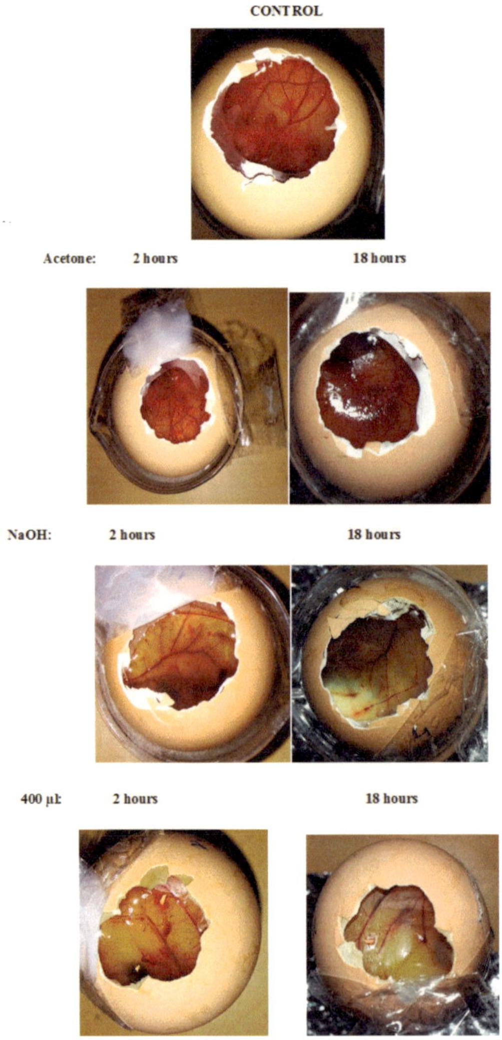

Figure 5. HET-CAM test on chick embryo control.

3.5. HET-CAM test on chick embryo

The CAM assay is a perceptive, easily feasible, and cheap in vivo check for enquiries of the anti-angiogenic promise of individual compounds. The compound TA4 inhibited the angiogenesis at an interval of 2 and 18 h (**Table 4** and **Figure 5**). This evinced that the compound has the good anti-angiogenic potentiality which could be explored as anticancer agents.

4. Discussion

In our current scenario there are many new and interesting bioactive metabolites applied as antibiotics, antiviral, anticancer and antioxidant compounds, which are of pharmaceutical, industrial and agricultural importance. Those have been investigated, reported and characterized from several fungal endophytes especially from medicinal plants/trees. Endophytic fungi have the ability to pulse up a plethora of secondary metabolites, typically dependent on the stage of development and environmental factors ranging from nutrient concentrations to light and temperature. The biosynthesis of pigmented secondary metabolite(s) is directly related to cultural conditions that include biomass in the production phase and duration of the incubation periods [14].

An investigation of Strobel and Daisy [15] suggested the endophytic fungi since such plants may harbor unique and rare endophytes capable of producing important bioactive metabolites with multiple applications. First and foremost pharmaceutical applied drug Taxol, an anticancer drug was derived from *Taxus*, a gymnosperm is an important anticancer plant. Several endophytic fungi isolated from *Taxus* spp., worldwide have been reported to produce important bioactive metabolites [16, 17]. This current investigation is focused to produce the pigmented crude secondary metabolites and purify a bioactive compound through the antioxidant assessment which could be taken for anticancer applications by *in vitro* and *in vivo* studies. The isolated and identified endophytic fungus FC36AY1 was a prospective and potential strain on analyzing antagonistic and preliminary antioxidant analysis. The fungus explored highest activity in both the assessment. The antagonism revealed the extent of this analysis ability increased as the endophytic fungal colonies matured when compared to immature colonies. The significant inhibition in the growth of fungi without direct contact of mycelia suggests that the prevailing antagonisms may be due to the production of inhibitory substances by the fungi or due to the competition for nutrients or both [18]. However, the mechanisms of inhibition in colony growth of the tested fungi were not addressed in our studies. This was similar to the investigation of Tayung et al. [17] investigated an endophytic fungus *Fusarium* sp. with highest antimicrobial and antioxidant analysis isolate from India. The potential strain was taken for the identification which showed up the organism was *Aspergillus terreus* FC36AY1 with the NCBI BankIt ID accession number was KY807648.

The study focused to produce the mass cultivation of pigmented crude secondary metabolites using SDB as production medium on which the strain FC36AY1 produced about 2.31 U/g in 1 L of production medium. The produced crude pigments were extracted using acetone as sole solvent from the fungal mat (biomass). This was similar to the study of Mani et al. [7] which explored that the extraction of pigmented secondary metabolites was done only in mid polar solvents. The crude pigmented metabolites were experimented for the purification process through HPLC analysis on which the crude was separated into 6 different fractions. Those fractions were taken for the assessment of antimicrobial and antioxidant activities. The 4th fraction TA4 was found to scavenge more free radicals at minimum concentration in a dose dependent manner and this was similar to the investigation of Samaga et al. [19]. In living organisms, oxidative stress created by reactive oxygen species (ROS) resulting from metabolism, in the form of superoxide anion (O^{-2}), hydroxyl radical (·OH), hydrogen peroxide (H_2O_2) and nitric oxide (NO) leads to conditions like cancer, stroke, myocardial infarctions, diabetes, septic and hemorrhagic shock, and neurodegenerative diseases by inducing biomolecular oxidations. Therefore, effective free radical scavenging molecules are needed by food and pharmaceutical industries. The fraction TA4 exhibited effective free radical scavenging activity comparable with that of BHA. The free radical scavenging activity of this particular fraction could be attributed to the presence of phenolic compounds [7]. This fraction was taken for the elucidation purpose through FT-IR and GC-MS analysis, on which TA4 showed similarity with 96–100% for the mass spectra of the compound and FT-IR exhibited the functional groups present in the compound and this was similar to the study of Liu et al. [11]. From this characterization, we found that the compound was octadecenoic acid 4-hydroxy methyl ester C19H38O3. This compound was taken for cytotoxicity analysis on HT-29 colon cancer cell lines, the compound TA4 explored its activity by showing a promising strategy of killing the cancer cells in an efficient manner. This was similar to the study of Devi and Prabakaran [20] in which they had experimented on four different cancer cell lines by using a potential bioactive compound from endophytic fungus.

The compound was taken for determination of anti-angiogenesis on chick embryo and this HET-CAM test exhibited maximum anti-angiogenesis by inhibiting maximum number of blood vessels. This manifesting that the compound TA4 has the ability to target the cancer cells and destruct by inhibiting the angiogenesis mechanism which is an important thing in oncology. The drug should have the ability to kill the cancer cells and also destruct the angiogenesis mechanism which could lead to metastasis i.e., taking the cancer cells to other parts of the body through the blood vessels and colonize in some particular area of the human body. In this case, we have found a potential bioactive compound from an efficient endophytic fungus possessing the ability to target the angiogenesis and avoid the metastasis. This is the first report that a bioactive compound TA4 from *A. terrus* FC36AY1 possessing the ability of anti-angiogenesis which was identified through HET-CAM analysis. From this investigation, we are concluding the compound TA4 evincing the ability to target the cancer cells and also it possess multi-functionality in medicinal fields.

5. Conclusion

The current scenario of the biotechnological research is searching for a new natural drug which could efficiently target on different diseases. This research mainly focuses on cancer study by isolating and characterizing a bioactive compound which exhibit its cytotoxicity and anti-angiogenesis against cancer cell lines. The compound TA4 manifested its characteristics by exploring its activities in different analysis. Finally, this investigation concludes that the compound TA4 has broad variety of bio-activities which emphasis in pharma and medicinal fields.

Conflict of interest

The authors declare that we do not have any conflict of interest.

Author details

Vellingiri Manon Mani[1,2*†], Arockiam Jeyasundar Parimala Gnana Soundari[2†] and Selvam Tamilarasi[1]

*Address all correspondence to: manonmanisathee12@gmail.com

1 PG and Research Department of Biotechnology, Hindusthan College of Arts and Science, Coimbatore, Tamil Nadu, India

2 Department of Microbial Biotechnology, Bharathiar University, Coimbatore, Tamil Nadu, India

† Both the authors contributed equally.

References

[1] Dufosse L. Pigments. Microbial Encyclopdic Microbiology. 2009;**4**:457-471

[2] Puri J. Endophytic fungi for producing bioactive compounds originally from their host plants. Cancer Chemotherapeutics Pharmacology. 2015;**44**:355-361

[3] Faeth RJ. Fungal Endophytes Diversity and Functional Roles. Tucson, AZ 85721, USA: University of Arizona; 2002

[4] Grube M, Cardinale M, de Castro JV, Müller H, Berg G. Species-specific structural and functional diversity of bacterial communities in lichen symbioses. The ISME Journal. 2009;**3**(9):1105-1115. DOI: 10.1038/ismej.2009.63

[5] Flewelling AJ, Ellsworth KT, Sanford J, Forward E, Johnson JA, Gray CA. Macroalgal endophytes from the Atlantic Coast of Canada: A potential source of antibiotic natural products. Microorganisms. 2013;**1**(1):175-187. DOI: 10.3390/microorganisms1010175

[6] Nassar AH. Activity of crude extracts of endophytic fungi isolated from medicinal plants. Australian Journal of Botany. 2005;**51**:257-266

[7] Mani VM, Soundari APG, Karthiyaini D, Preethi K. Bioprospecting for endophytic fungi and their metabolites from medicinal tree *Aegle marmelos* in Western Ghats, India. Mycobiology. 2015;**43**(3):303-310

[8] Wiener B. F. Geiss. Fundamentals of thin layer chromatography planar chromatography. Heidelberg, Dr. A. Hüthig Verlag, 1987, 482 S., 202 Abb., 40 Tab., DM 192,–, ISBN 3-7785-0854-7. Acta Hydrochimica et Hydrobiologica Banner. 1997;**16**:653. DOI: 10.1002/aheh.19880160622

[9] Oyaizu M. Studies on product of browning reaction prepared from glucoseamine. Japanese Journal of Nutrition. 1986;**44**:307-315

[10] Dinis TCP, Madeira VMC, Almeida LM. Action of phenolic derivates (acetoaminophen, salycilate and 5-aminosalycilate) as inhibitors of membrane lipid peroxidation and as peroxyl radical scavengers. Journal of Archives in Biochemistry and Biophysics. 1994;**315**:161-169

[11] Liu X, Dong M, Chen X, Jiang M, Lv X, Zhou J. Antimicrobial activity of an endophytic *Xylaria* sp. YX-28 and identification of its antimicrobial compound 7-amino-4-methylcoumarin. Applied Microbiology and Biotechnology. 2008;**78**:241-247

[12] Yu W, Zhao Y, Shu B. The radical scavenging activities of radix puerariae isoflavonoids: A chemiluminescence study. Food Chemistry. 2004;**86**:525

[13] Yuvaraj N, Kanmani P, Satishkumar R, Paari KA, Pattukuma V, Arul V. Extraction, purification and partial characterization of *Cladophora glomerata* against multidrug resistant human pathogen, *Acinetobacter baumannii* and fish pathogens. World Journal of Fisheries and Marine Sciences. 2011;**3**:51-57

[14] Pradeep FS, Pradeep BV. Optimization of pigment and biomass production from *Fusarium moniliforme* under submerged fermentation conditions. International Journal of Pharmacy and Pharmaceutical Sciences. 2013;**5**(3):526-535

[15] Strobel G, Daisy D. Bioprospecting for microbial endophytes and their natural products. Microbiology and Molecular Biology Reviews. 2003;**67**:491-502. DOI: 10.1128/MMBR.67.4.491-502.2003

[16] Wang HS, Lu Y, Xue Y, Ruan ZY, Jiang RB, Xing XH, et al. Separation, purification and structure identification of purple pigments from *Dunaliella* sp. B2. Journal of Chemistry and Industrial Engineering. 2008;**59**:630-635

[17] Tayung K, Barik BP, Jagadev PN, Mohapatra UB. Phylogenetic investigation of endophytic *Fusarium* strain producing antimicrobial metabolite isolated from Himalayan Yew Bark. Malaysian Journal of Microbiology. 2011;**7**:1-6. DOI: 10.21161/mjm.23810

[18] Powthong P, Thongmee A, Suntornthiticharoen P. Antioxidant and antimicrobial activities of endophytic fungi isolated from *Sesbania grandiflora* (l.) pers. International Journal of Phytomedicine. 2013;**5**(1):102-107

[19] Samaga PV, Rai VR, Rai KML. *Bionectria ochroleuca* NOTL33—An endophytic fungus from Nothapodytes foetida producing antimicrobial and free radical scavenging metabolites. Annals of Microbiology. 2013;**13**:661-666

[20] Devi NN, Prabakaran JJ. Bioactive metabolites from an endophytic fungus Penicillium sp isolated from *Centella asciatica*. Current Research in Environment and Applied Mycology. 2014;**4**(1):34-43

Chapter 3

The Apoptotic Effects of Methylparaben and Ultraviolet B Light on M624 Human Melanoma Cells

Rebekah S. Wood, Rebecca S. Greenstein,
Isabella M. Hildebrandt and
Kimberly S. George Parsons

Additional information is available at the end of the chapter

http://dx.doi.org/10.5772/intechopen.78575

Abstract

Methylparaben is a commonly used antimicrobial in cosmetics that has been shown to have negative effects on mammalian cells. Human melanoma M624 cells were treated with 1 and 5 mM methylparaben in the presence and absence of 25 mJ/cm^2 ultraviolet B (UV-B) light. Cell proliferation assays showed that 5 mM methylparaben was toxic to M624 cells after 24 hours. Apoptotic signaling pathways were analyzed via isolation of separate cellular compartments and protein analysis via western blot. Upon 5 mM methylparaben treatment, PARP I was cleaved indicating apoptosis, which was mediated by the TNF-α receptor activated in the lipid rafts of the M624 cells. Upon 25 mJ/cm^2 UV-B radiation, PARP II was activated indicating cellular damage, cytochrome c was released from the mitochondria, and caspase-3 was expressed. Upon combinatory treatment with 5 mM methylparaben and 25 mJ/cm^2 UV-B, apoptosis was induced through mitochondrial release of cytochrome c, expression of caspase-3 and cleavage of PARP I, while methylparaben-induced TNF-α receptor activation and UV-B-induced PARP II activation was inhibited., demonstrating that antimicrobial methylparaben in cosmetics can cause damage to cells.

Keywords: methylparaben, ultraviolet light, apoptosis

1. Introduction

Paraben compounds are antimicrobials used in cosmetics as preservatives due to their broad antimicrobial functions and their ability to meet the criteria for an ideal preservative [1].

However, the side effects of paraben use include increased estrogenic activity of receptors, sensitization of broken skin, endocrine disruptive effects and adverse reproductive effects [2]. The paraben group of compounds includes methyl, ethyl, butyl, heptyl, and benzyl parabens. Methylparaben, a methylester of *p*-hydroxybenzoic acid, is the most widely used paraben in topical skin products [3]. Studies have recently shown that small amounts of methylparaben remain unhydrolyzed in the epidermis [4]. Handa et al. has been the first to describe the effects of methylparaben and ultraviolet B (UV-B) radiation as detrimental to human skin HaCaT keratinocytes [3].

Handa et al. studied HaCaT keratinocytes treated with UV-B and methylparaben. HaCaT keratinocytes were cultured in methylparaben-containing medium concentrations of 19.7, 1.97, and 0.197 mM (0.3, 0.03, and 0.003%) for 24 hours, exposed to UV-B (15 or 30 mJ/cm^2) and further cultured for another 24 hours. The use of parabens in cosmetic products is permitted up to 0.8% (w/w), however the concentration in cosmetics is typically less than 0.32% [4]. Cellular viability, cell death, oxidative stress, nitric oxide production, cellular lipid peroxidation, and activation of nuclear factor kappa B and activator protein-1 were studied, demonstrating that methylparaben treatment increases cell death when the cells are exposed to UV-B and that the detrimental potential of methylparaben is dose and time dependent [3].

Ultraviolet B radiation (290–320 nm) is the main cause of tumor initiation and promotion [5]. UV-B is 1000 times more likely than UVA to cause sunburn and is also known to cause melanoma: while some of the harmful UV-B rays are absorbed by the ozone layer, some still penetrate the atmosphere, causing sunburns that lead to skin cancer.

Melanoma is the deadliest of the skin cancers and accounts for approximately three fourths of all skin cancer deaths [6]. Forms of melanoma currently being diagnosed and treated include superficial spreading melanoma (most common), lentigo maligna, lentiginous melanoma and nodular melanoma. The mechanism for UV-B-induced cancer can be attributed to the dysregulation of apoptosis, or programmed cell death. Apoptosis is a fundamental mechanism characterized by cell shrinkage, membrane blebbing, nuclear breakdown, and DNA fragmentation that is needed for embryonic development, tissue homeostasis, immune defense, and elimination of harmful cells [7]. Ultimately, the cell and its contents are broken down to membrane bound fragments that are phagocytosed by adjacent cells [8]. The apoptotic pathway is regulated by death receptor-mediated extrinsic pathways and mitochondria-mediated intrinsic pathways [9]. The dysregulation of apoptosis can result in pathophysiological states and diseases, such as cancer [7]. Dysregulation in the UV-B-induced apoptosis may also have a major impact on photocarcinogenesis [10].

The PARP protein is an indicator of apoptosis. PARP I cleavage is an indication of induced apoptosis, while PARP II expression is an indicator of advanced cellular damage. PARP I and PARP II are activated by DNA interruptions and are involved in cell survival/death, transcription, DNA repair, and cell division [11, 12]. They act as both damage sensors and signal transducers to down-stream effectors [11, 13]. PARP I and PARP II also function to signal the cell to undergo apoptosis when the amount of DNA damage is beyond repair capacity [13]. PARP I will cleave into 89- and 24-kDa fragments that contain the active site and the DNA-binding domain of the enzyme during apoptosis. The caspase cascade is an important apoptotic signaling pathway, and caspase-3 is known to be responsible for the cleavage of PARP I during cell death. The sequence at which caspase-3 cleaves PARP I is well conserved in distant species, indicating an important role for PARP I cleavage in apoptosis [14].

One major regulator of apoptosis is the mitochondria through release of apoptotic factors, such as cytochrome c, through permeabilization of the outer mitochondrial membrane. The rapid increase in permeability causes depolarization, uncoupling of oxidative phosphorylation, and mitochondrial swelling [8]. The mitochondrial pathway of apoptosis through the mitochondrial permeability transition is important for the elimination of UV-B-damaged human keratinocytes [15]. Cytochrome c is a soluble protein that participates in the electron transfer between complex III and complex IV of the respiratory chain in a normal functioning cell [16]. However, an apoptotic signal can lead to the release of cytochrome c from the intermembrane space of the mitochondria into the cytosol. Cells undergoing apoptosis may have an elevation of cytochrome c in the cytosol and a corresponding decrease in the mitochondria [17]. Once released, cytochrome c can bind to the adaptor molecule apoptotic protease activating factor-1 (Apaf-1) and can subsequently activate caspase-9 or caspase-8. Finally, caspase-3 can be activated which is the irreversible point in the mitochondrial apoptosis pathway [9].

Another important regulator of apoptotic induction in the cell is contents of the lipid raft domains. Lipid rafts contain plasma membrane proteins compartmentalized into sphingolipid- and cholesterol-rich microdomains and function as platforms for signal transduction [18]. These lipid raft domains are dynamic, float freely within the bilayer and coalesce upon clustering of their components [19]. Sphingolipids and cholesterol are necessary for the assembly of the lipid raft compartments [20]. Lipid rafts and associated proteins are known to be important in the pathogenesis of several diseases, including cancer progression. In the lipid rafts, caveolin-1 functions through direct protein–protein interactions to regulate diverse cellular processes, including raft-mediated endocytosis, vesicular transport, cell migration, and signal transduction [21]. An upregulation of caveolin-1 expression in clinical studies was associated with the occurrence of metastasis [22]. Caveolin-1 is a lipid raft indicator protein because it is a cholesterol binding protein. This is important because the integrity of the lipid raft is dependent on the ability of cholesterol to pack tightly with the saturated sphingolipids [23]. TNF-α binds to the TNF receptor (TNFR) to initiate apoptosis [24]. TNF-α is a pleiotropic cytokine that can signal for proliferation, stress, inflammation, and cell death [8]. The TNF pathway occurs in a number of different cell types [25]. Cytochrome c is located downstream in the tumor necrosis factor α (TNF-α) apoptotic pathway.

While Handa et al. demonstrated the apoptotic effects of methylparaben in normal skin cells, this study examines the apoptotic signaling pathways activated by methylparaben in cancerous melanoma cells, as well as the role (or absence of role) of the mitochondria and lipid raft domains in these signaling pathways. In this study, we have analyzed the expression and activation of the nuclear apoptotic indicator PARP I, PARP II, and cleaved PARP proteins, as well as the expression of TNF-α receptor in the lipid rafts in UV-B and methylparaben-treated human M624 melanoma cells. In addition, the expression of caspase-3 and the expression and location of cytochrome c were also analyzed under these cellular conditions in order to fully characterize the cell signaling pathway activated by the cosmetic antimicrobial agent methylparaben.

2. Materials and methods

2.1. Cell culture and treatment

Transformed M624 human melanoma cells were obtained from Dr. Shiyong Wu's laboratory (Edison Biotechnology Institute, Ohio University, Ohio, USA) and originally generated by the National Institute of Health (NIH) (USA). Cells were cultured in DMEM supplemented with fetal bovine serum (FBS) (10%) and penicillin/streptomycin (1%). At 80% cell confluency, cells were treated with methylparaben and UV-B. Cells were incubated with 1 or 5 mM methylparaben in media including supplements for 2 hours. The methylparaben media was removed while treating the cells with 25 mJ/cm^2 UV-B radiation and replaced after radiation, and then incubated for another 4 hours before cell lysis.

2.2. Cell proliferation assays

Cells were plated at approximately 25% confluency and then treated with methylparaben and UV-B radiation as described above, except paraben solutions were allowed to incubate for 24 hours and then viable cells were stained using 0.5% crystal violet solution. Results are averaged from three independent trials.

2.3. Protein samples

Whole Cell Lysate Preparation Cells were washed three times with cold, 1X Phosphate Buffered Saline (PBS) (10 mM phosphate). Cells were then placed in a −20°C freezer for at least 2 hours, removed, and washed once more with PBS. TNET lysis buffer (25 mM Tris–HCl pH 7.5, 150 mM NaCl, 5 mM EDTA, and 0.1% Triton X-100) was mixed with protease inhibitors and added to the cells. The solution containing cells was homogenized with 23 gauge needles and syringes and centrifuged at low speed after which supernatant was collected.

2.4. Lipid raft isolation

Lipid rafts were prepared as previously described [26]. Briefly, 3,3′-dithiobis (sulfosuccinimidyl propionate) (DTSSP) (1.25 m M) was added to each plate of cells after UV-B and methylparaben treatment and incubated for 1 hour at 4°C. The cells were then collected and frozen overnight. Cells were washed and lysed as described above to prepare samples and placed in an iodixanol solution gradient and ultra-centrifuged for 5 hours. Fractions were collected and the lipid rafts were present in fraction two, indicated by the presence of caveolin-1 protein.

2.5. Mitochondrial isolation

Cells were washed with PBS and suspended in an isotonic buffer (10 mM Hepes, pH 7.4, 0.2 M mannitol, 0.07 M sucrose) supplemented with protease inhibitors. Samples were homogenized and then centrifuged at 900× g for 5 minutes. Then cells were centrifuged at 10,000× g for 30 minutes at 4°C to obtain the heavy membrane pellet. Samples were re-suspended in an SEM buffer (250 mM Sucrose, 1 mM EDTA, 10 mM MOPS-KOH, pH 7.2).

2.6. Sample preparation

Samples were prepared by adding protein loading buffer (0.25 M Tris, pH 6.8, 10% sodium dodecyl sulfate, 0.05% bromophenol blue, 50% glycerol, 10 mM β-mercaptoethanol). The samples were vortexed, boiled for 5 minutes, vortexed and then stored at −20°C.

2.7. SDS-page

SDS-PAGE was performed using a 15% separating gel and 4% stacking gel to create a gel with 1.0 mm thickness. Protein samples were separated at 200 volts for 45 minutes and then transferred to a nitrocellulose membrane via wet transfer at 100 volts for 35 minutes. After the transfer, the nitrocellulose membrane was blocked using dried non-fat milk in 1× tris buffered saline with 0.05% Tween (TBS-T) for 20 minutes.

2.8. Western blot

Western blot was performed using β-actin primary antibody (122 M4782, Sigma, St. Louis, MO) for 3 hours followed by three rinse wash cycles and then probed with anti-mouse secondary antibody (Santa Cruz Biotechnology, sc-2371) for 1 hour. PARP protein expression and cleavage was detected by probing overnight with PARP primary antibody (MA5–15031, Thermo Fisher Scientific, Waltham, MA) and anti-rabbit secondary antibody (32,260, Thermo Fisher Scientific, Waltham, MA). Caveolin-1 protein expression was detected by probing overnight with caveolin-1 primary antibody (sc-894, Santa Cruz Biotechnology, Dallas, TX) and anti-rabbit secondary antibody. TNF R1 protein expression was detected by probing overnight with TNF R1 primary antibody (sc-7418, Santa Cruz Biotechnology, Dallas, TX) and anti-mouse secondary antibody. Cytochrome c protein expression was detected by probing with cytochrome c HRP-conjugated primary antibody (sc-13,156, Santa Cruz Biotechnology, Dallas, TX) overnight. Caspase-3 protein expression was detected by probing overnight with Caspase-3 primary antibody (sc-7418, Santa Cruz Biotechnology, Dallas, TX) and anti-rabbit secondary antibody. All overnight incubations were performed shaking at 5°C; all other incubations were performed shaking at room temperature. Protein expression was visualized via chemiluminescence (SuperSignal West Pico Chemiluminescent Substrate).

3. Results

The toxicity of methylparaben and UV-B light to human melanoma M624 cells was initially analyzed using a clonogenic cell proliferation assay (**Figure 1**). The effects of methylparaben and UV-B light on apoptotic pathways in M624 cells were then investigated by analyzing expression of PARP and caspase-3 and cleavage of PARP in the whole cell lysate samples, TNF-α expression in the lipid rafts, and cytochrome c expression in both mitochondrial and regular lysate samples, via SDS-PAGE and western blot (**Figures 2–4**).

Human M624 melanoma cells were treated with methylparaben (1 and 5 mM) and 25 mJ/cm^2 UV-B. The 5 mM concentration of methylparaben and the 25 mJ/cm^2 UV-B were each shown

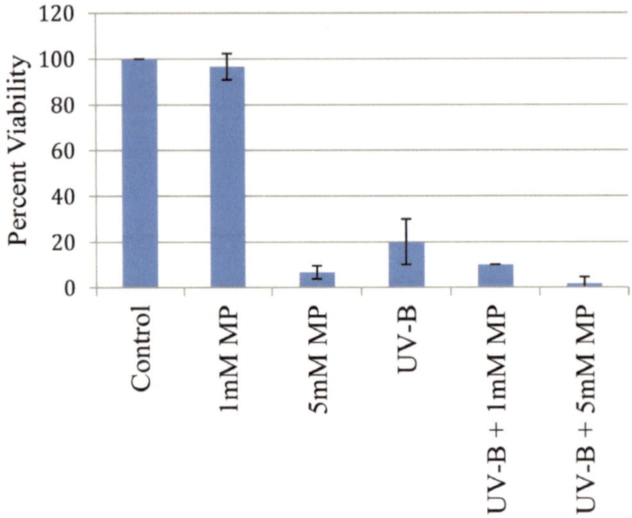

Figure 1. Phototoxicity studies: Crystal violet proliferative assay: cells were treated with methylparaben and UV-B radiation and then stained with a 0.5% crystal violet solution after 24 hours.

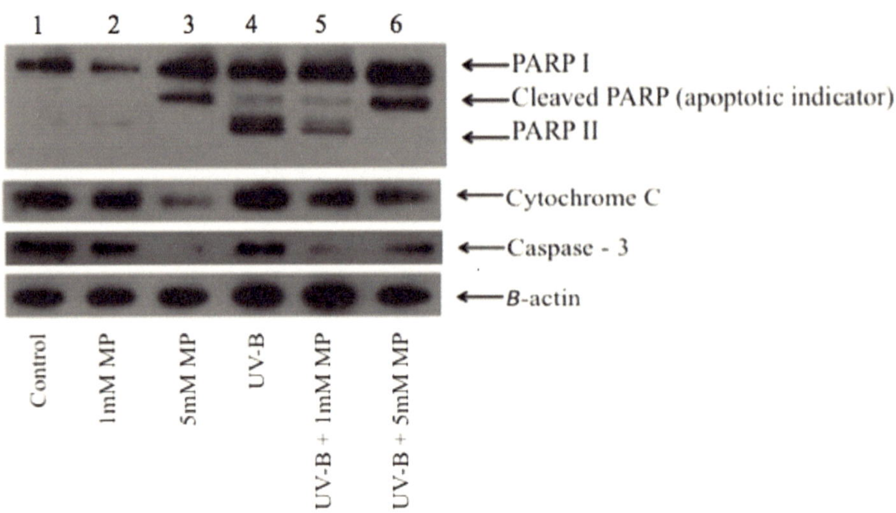

Figure 2. Western blot of whole cell lysate protein samples of PARP I, and cleaved PARP I, PARP II, cytochrome c and caspase 3. Samples were standardized using β-actin western blot.

to be toxic to the M624 human melanoma cells after 24 hours (**Figure 1**). The combination of methylparaben treatment and UV-B radiation showed amplified toxicity, even at the 1 mM paraben concentration level after 24 hours; 1 mM methylparaben alone was nontoxic to the cells (**Figure 1**).

Results showed that 5 mM methylparaben induced PARP I cleavage (lane 3), while 25 mJ/cm^2 UV-B induced PARP II expression instead (lane 4). When cells were treated with UV-B and

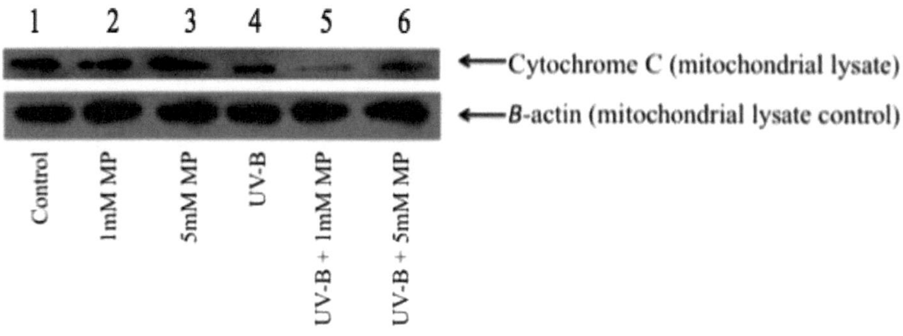

Figure 3. Western blot of mitochondrial protein samples of cytochrome c. Samples were standardized using β-actin western blot.

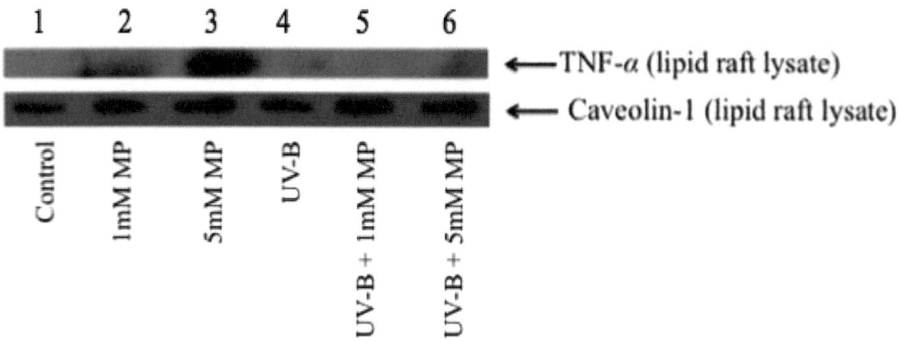

Figure 4. Western blot of lipid raft protein samples of TNF-α. Samples were standardized using caveolin-1 western blot.

5 mM methylparaben, UV-B-induced PARP II expression was completely inhibited (lane 6) while UV-B and 1 mM methylparaben partially inhibited the PARP II expression. Overall, methylparaben at 5 mM had an impact on PARP cleavage with and without UV-B and was able to inhibit UV-B-induced PARP II expression (**Figure 2**).

Cytochrome c protein expression in the whole cell and mitochondrial lysate samples was analyzed using β-actin standardized loading amounts. Cytochrome c expression was reduced in the whole cell lysate samples treated with 5 mM methylparaben and 5 mM methylparaben plus UV-B (**Figure 2**, lanes 3 and 6 versus lane 1) while cytochrome c expression in the mitochondrial lysate 5 mM methylparaben sample was relatively unchanged compared to the expression seen in the control mitochondrial lysate sample (**Figure 3**, lane 3 versus lane 1). UV-B radiation caused a decrease in cytochrome c in the mitochondrial samples treated with or without methylparaben (**Figure 3**, lanes 4, 5 and 6 versus lane 1).

Caspase-3 expression was analyzed in whole cell lysate samples using β-actin standardized loading amounts. It was shown that caspase-3 expression was decreased when the M624 human melanoma cells were treated with 5 mM methylparaben, 1 mM methylparaben plus UV-B radiation, and 5 mM methylparaben plus UV-B radiation when compared to the control sample (**Figure 2**, lanes 3, 5 and 6 versus lane 1). On the other hand, caspase-3 expression was greater in the sample treated with UV-B radiation when combined with 5 mM methylparaben treatment compared to 5 mM methylparaben treatment alone (**Figure 2**, lane 6 versus lane 3).

After standardizing the lipid raft samples via caveolin-1, TNF-α receptor expression in the lipid raft fraction was analyzed. Western blot analysis revealed that the expression of TNF-α receptor was increased in the cells treated with 5 mM of methylparaben compared with control cells (**Figure 4**, lane 3 versus lane 1). This methylparaben-induced increase in expression was inhibited in cells treated with UV-B light (**Figure 4**, lane 6 versus lane 3).

4. Discussion

Melanoma is the deadliest of the skin cancers and accounts for approximately three fourths of all skin cancer deaths [6]. Previous research performed by Handa et al. has shown the detrimental effects of methylparaben and UV-B treatment on HaCaT cells [3]. This study is the first to demonstrate the effects of methylparaben and UV-B in M624 human melanoma cells.

Phototoxicity studies performed on M624 human melanoma cells have shown that 5 mM methylparaben is toxic to M624 cells and UV-B exposure increases this toxicity (**Figure 1**). The PARP protein is an indicator of apoptosis: DNA interruptions activate PARP I and PARP II; PARP I cleavage is an indicator that apoptosis has been induced and PARP II expression is an indicator of cellular damage. PARP I and PARP II function to signal the cell to undergo apoptosis when the amount of DNA damage is beyond the repair capacity [13]. Results indicate that apoptosis occurred after 5 mM methylparaben and 5 mM methylparaben plus UV-B treatment due to the increased cleavage of PARP I. PARP II expression was induced after 25 mJ/cm^2 UV-B treatment indicated cellular damage. UV-B-induced PARP II expression was partially inhibited in the cells treated with 1 mM methylparaben and completely inhibited in the cells treated with 5 mM methylparaben, indicating that PARP II is not involved in the signaling pathway activated by 5 mM methylparaben in combination with UV-B radiation and that methylparaben-induced apoptosis is concentration-dependent (**Figure 2**).

Since cleavage of PARP I indicates that apoptosis was occurring in cells treated with methylparaben, and activation of PARP II indicates cellular damage was occurring in cells treated with methylparaben and UV-B radiation, the involvement of the mitochondria and the lipid rafts in the signaling pathways was then analyzed.

The apoptotic signal can be propagated through an intrinsic mitochondrial response that causes permeabilization of the outer mitochondrial membrane in order to release cytochrome c into the cytosol [7]. Analysis of cytochrome c in both whole cell and mitochondrial isolated samples enabled determination of the movement of cytochrome c under different treatment conditions. Most notably, there were changes in cytochrome c expression in the cells treated with 5 mM methylparaben compared to the cells treated with UV-B light radiation with or without methylparaben. In the 5 mM methylparaben treated sample, cytochrome c expression remained unchanged in the mitochondrial lysate while there was decreased expression of

http://dx.doi.org/10.5772/intechopen.78575

cytochrome c in the whole cell lysate sample upon 5 mM methylparaben treatment indicating no release of cytochrome c from the mitochondria in these cells. On the other hand, UV-B light treatment showed a decreased cytochrome c expression in the mitochondrial isolated sample while the whole cell lysate sample showed an increased or unchanged cytochrome c expression in cells treated with or without methylparaben indicating a UV-B-induced apoptotic release of cytochrome c from the mitochondria.

The same pattern of expression was seen with caspase-3, indicating caspase-3 activation upon release of cytochrome c from the mitochondria in cells treated with UV-B and UV-B with 5 mM methylparaben. However, 5 mM methylparaben treatment alone inhibited caspase-3 expression. These results suggest that both UV-B light and UV-B light radiation in addition to the 5 mM methylparaben treatment results in M624 human melanoma cells taking a different apoptotic pathway in comparison to cell treatment with only 5 mM methylparaben. When human melanoma M624 cells are exposed to UV-B light or both 5 mM methylparaben and UV-B light, apoptosis occurs through the intrinsic pathway as indicated with the release of cytochrome c from the mitochondria and expression of caspase-3. In comparison, treatment with only 5 mM methylparaben does not result in the release of cytochrome c from the mitochondria into the cytosol or caspase-3 expression (**Figures 2** and **3**).

The TNF-α receptor expression in the lipid rafts of M624 melanoma cells induced by methylparaben and UV-B radiation was analyzed by western blot analysis of lipid raft samples. Results show that apoptosis was initiated through the TNF-α receptor when treated with 5 mM methylparaben, but the involvement of the TNF-α receptor was inhibited in the presence of UV-B light. The integrity of the lipid raft is dependent on the ability of cholesterol to pack tightly with the saturated sphingolipids [23]. Caveolin-1 in the lipid rafts binds to cholesterol, which is necessary for the assembly of the lipid raft components [20]. Caveolin-1 expression was used to standardize the lipid raft samples in order to examine the expression of the TNF-α receptor in the lipid rafts of cells. TNF-α commonly initiates apoptosis by binding to the TNF-α receptor [24]. The activation of TNF-α receptor can lead to formation of TNFR1-associated death domain protein (TRADD). TRADD recruits Fas-associated protein with death domain (FADD) and leads to caspase activation and apoptosis [27]. Death domain formation occurs only when TNF-α receptor is translocated into lipid raft domains [19]; therefore, the expression of the receptor in the lipid rafts was analyzed. Results showed expression of TNF-α receptor in the lipid rafts of cells treated with 5 mM methylparaben, which was inhibited in the presence of UV-B radiation (**Figure 4**). These results suggest an alternate TNF-α apoptotic pathway that does not involve the release of cytochrome c from the mitochondria into the cytosol or expression of caspase-3.

TNF-α apoptotic pathways exist that do not cause the release of cytochrome c from the mitochondria that should be investigated in future studies. One of these TNF-α apoptotic pathway involves inhibition of NF-κB to allow JNK to induce caspase 8-independent cleavage of Bid to produce jBid. jBid then translocates into the mitochondria to induce the release of Smac, but not cytochrome c. [27, 28]. This research and future steps in this project are important to the understanding of the apoptotic pathway in human M624 melanoma cells when treated with methylparaben and UV-B radiation.

5. Conclusion

This study has demonstrated cell damage, cellular apoptosis and cellular damage upon exposure to the cosmetic antimicrobial methylparaben. In summary, results show that upon 5 mM methylparaben treatment, PARP I was cleaved indicating apoptosis, which was mediated by the TNF-α receptor activated in the lipid rafts of the M624 cells (**Figure 5a**). Upon 25 mJ/cm^2

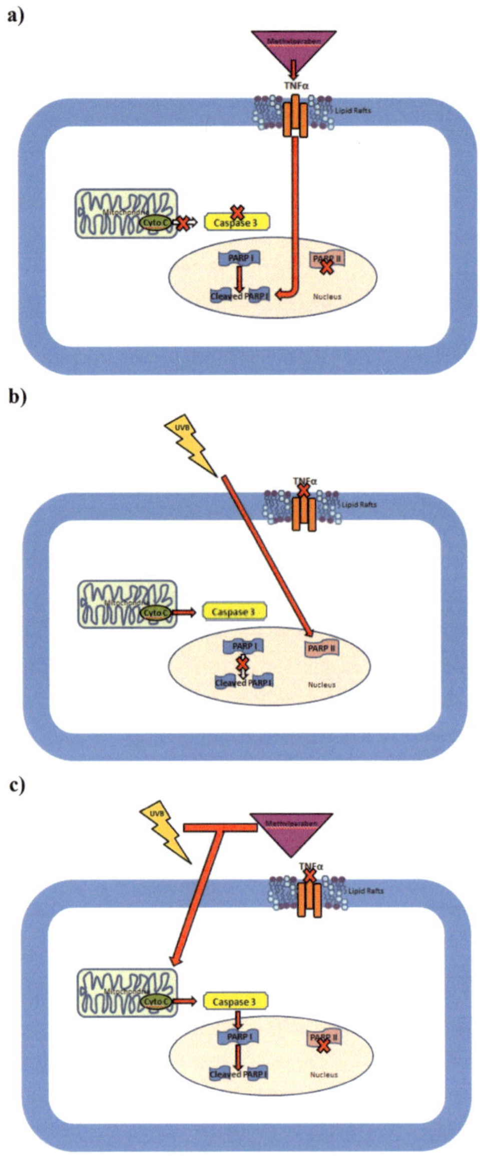

Figure 5. Apoptotic pathways: (a) apoptotic proteins activated by 5 mM methylparaben; (b) apoptotic proteins activated by 25 mJ/cm^2 UV-B; (c) apoptotic proteins activated by combination of 5 mM methylparaben and 25 mJ/cm^2 UV-B.

UV-B radiation, PARP II was activated indicating cellular damage, cytochrome c was released from the mitochondria, and caspase-3 was expressed in the cell (**Figure 5b**). Upon combinatory treatment with 5 mM methylparaben and 25 mJ/cm^2 UV-B, apoptosis was induced through mitochondrial release of cytochrome c, expression of caspase-3 (and the caspase cascade) and cleavage of PARP I (**Figure 5c**). Differences in signaling pathways treated with 1 versus 5 mM methylparaben suggest concentration-dependent activation of apoptosis in M624 cells. Future studies will further elucidate the details of the signaling pathways through analysis of additional apoptotic proteins and lipids of the cells.

Acknowledgements

Thank you to Dr. Shiyong Wu's lab for donation of cells. Thanks to the Departments of Chemistry and Biochemistry and Biology of Marietta College for all funding for this project.

Conflict of interest

No conflicts of interest.

Author details

Rebekah S. Wood[1], Rebecca S. Greenstein[2], Isabella M. Hildebrandt[3] and Kimberly S. George Parsons[4]*

*Address all correspondence to: ksg001@marietta.edu

1 Boonshoft School of Medicine, Wright State University, Dayton, Ohio, USA

2 University of Cincinnati College of Medicine, Cincinnati, Ohio, USA

3 College of Veterinary Medicine, Ohio State University, Columbus, Ohio, USA

4 Marietta College, Marietta, Ohio, USA

References

[1] Pugazhendhi D, Pope GS, Darbre PD. Oestrogenic activity of p-hydroxybenzoic acid (common metabolite of paraben esters) and methylparaben in human breast cancer cell lines. Journal of Applied Toxicology. 2005;**25**:301-309. DOI: 10.1002/jat.1066

[2] Cabaleiro N, Calle I, Bendich C, Lavilla I. An overview of sample preparation for the determination of parabens in cosmetics. Trends in Analytical Chemistry. 2014;**57**:34-46. DOI: 10.1016/j.trac.2014.02.003

[3] Handa O, Kokura S, Adachi S, Takagi T, Naito Y, Tanigawa T, Yoshida N, Yoshikawa T. Methylparaben potentiates UV-induced damage of skin keratinocytes. Toxicology. 2006;**22**:62-72. DOI: 10.1016/j.tox.2006.07.018

[4] Cross SE, Roberts MS. The effect of occlusion on epidermal penetration of parabens from a commercial allergy test ointment, acetone and ethanol vehicles. The Journal of Investigative Dermatology. 2000;**115**:914-918. DOI: 10.1046/j.1523-1747.2000.00151.x

[5] Buckman S, Gresham A, Hale P, Hruza G, Anast J, Masferrer J, Pentland A. COX-2 expression is induced by UV-B exposure in human skin: Implications for the development of skin cancer. Carcinogenesis. 1998;**19**:723-729

[6] Hall I, Miller D, Rogers J, Bewerse B. Update on the incidence and mortality from melanoma in the United States. Journal of the American Academy of Dermatology. 1999;**40**:35-42. DOI: 10.1016/S0190-9622(99)70562-1

[7] Yin H, Zhow Y, Zhu M, Hou S, Li Z, Zhong H, Lu J, Meng T, Wang J, Xia L, Xu Y, Wu Y. Role of mitochondria in programmed cell death mediated by arachidonic acid-derivedeicosanoids. Mitochondrion. 2013;**13**:209-224. DOI: 10.1016/j.mito.2012.10.003

[8] Bradham C, Qian T, Streetz K, Trautwein C, Brenner D, Lemasters J. The mitochondrial permeability transition is required for tumor necrosis factor alpha-mediated apoptosis and cytochrome c release. Molecular and Cellular Biology. 1998;**18**:6353-6364. DOI: 10.1128/MCB.18.11.6353

[9] Li W, Huang Y, Zhao X, Zhang W, Dong F, Du Q, Tong D. Swainsonine induces caprine luteal cells apoptosis via mitochondrial-mediated caspase-dependent pathway. Journal of Biochemical and Molecular Toxicology. 2014;**28**:456-464. DOI: 10.1002/jbt.21585

[10] Kulms D, Zeise E, Poppelmann B, Schwarz T. DNA damage, death receptor activation and reactive oxygen species contribute to ultraviolet radiation-induced apoptosis in an essential and independent way. Oncogene. 2002;**21**:5844-5851. DOI: 10.1038/sj.onc.1205743

[11] Yelamos J, Farres J, Llacuna L, Ampurdanes C, Martin-Caballero J. PARP-1 and PARP-2: New players in tumour development. American Journal of Cancer Research. 2011;**1**:328-346

[12] Geng B, Cai Y, Gao S, Lu J, Zhang L, Zou J, Liu M, Yu S, Ye J, Liu P. PARP-2 knockdown protects cardiomyocytes from hypertrophy via activation of SIRT1. Biochemical and Biophysical Research Communications. 2013;**3**:944-950. DOI: 10.1016/j.bbrc.2012.11.132

[13] Sousa F, Matuo R, Soares D, Escargueil E, Henriques J, Larsen A, Saffi J. PARPS and the DNA damage response. Carcinogenesis. 2012;**33**:1433-1440. DOI: 10.1093/carcin/bgs132

[14] Boulares A, Yakovlev A, Ivanova V, Stoica B, Wang G, Iyer S, Smulson M. Role of poly(ADP-ribose) polymerase (PARP) cleavage in apoptosis. The Journal of Biological Chemistry. 1999;**274**:22932-22940. DOI: 10.1074/jbc.274.33.22932

[15] Laethem A, Kelst S, Lippens S, Declercq W, Vandenabeele P, Janssens S, Vandenheede J, Garmyn M, Agostinis P. Activation of p38 MAPK is required for Bax translocation to

mitochondria, cytochrome c release and apoptosis induced by UV-B radiation in human keratinocytes. The FASEB Journal. 2004;**18**:1946-1978. DOI: 10.1096/fj.04-2285fje

[16] Seye C, Knaapen M, Daret D, Desgranges C, Herman A, Knockx M, Bult H. 7-Ketocholesterol induces reversible cytochrome c release in small muscle cells in absence of mitochondrial swelling. Cardiovascular Research. 2004;**64**:144-153

[17] Yang J, Liu X, Bhalla K, Kim C, Ibrado A, Cai J. Prevention of apoptosis by Bcl-2 release of cytochrome c from mitochondria blocked. Science. 1997;**275**:1129-1132. DOI: 10.1126/science.275.5303.1129

[18] Pike LJ. Lipid rafts: Heterogeneity on the high seas. The Biochemical Journal. 2004; **378**:281-292. DOI: 10.1042/bj20031672

[19] George KS, Wu S. Lipid raft: A floating island of death or survival. Toxicology and Applied Pharmacology. 2012;**15**:311-319. DOI: 10.1016/j.taap.2012.01.007

[20] Rajendran L, Simons K. Lipid rafts and membrane dynamics. Journal of Cell Science. 2005;**118**:1099-1102. DOI: 10.1242/jcs.01681

[21] Zhuang L, Kim J, Adam R, Soloman K, Freeman M. Cholesterol targeting alters lipid raft composition and cell survival in prostate cancer cells and xenografts. The Journal of Clinical Investigation. 2005;**115**:959-968. DOI: 10.1172/JCI19935

[22] Yamaguchi H, Takeo Y, Yoshida S, Kouchi Z, Nakamura Y, Fukami K. Lipid rafts and caveolin-1 are required for invadopodia formation and extracellular matrix degradation by human breast cancer cells. Cancer Research. 2009;**69**:8594-8602. DOI: 10.1158/0008-5472.CAN-09-2305

[23] Yu C, Alterman M, Dobrowsky R. Ceramide displaces cholesterol from lipid rafts and decreases the association of the cholesterol binding protein caveolin-1. Journal of Lipid Research. 2005;**46**:1678-1691. DOI: 10.1194/jlr.M500060-JLR200

[24] Wang C, Mayo M, Korneluk R, Goeddel D, Baldwin A. NF-κB Antiapoptosis: Induction of TRAF1 and TRAF2 and c-IAP1 and c-IAP2 to suppress caspase-8 activation. Science 1998;**281**:1680-1683

[25] Guicciardi M, Deussing J, Miyoshi H, Bronk S, Svingen P, Peters C, Kaufmann S, Gores G. Cathepsin B contributes to TNF-α-mediated hepatocyte apoptosis by promoting mitochondrial release of cytochrome c. The Journal of Clinical Investigation. 2000;**106**:1127-1137

[26] George K, Wu Q, Wu S. Effects of freezing and protein crosslinker on isolating membrane raft associated proteins. BioTechniques. 2010;**49**:837-838. DOI: 10.2144/000113541

[27] Deng Y, Ren X, Yang L, Lin Y, Wu X. A JNK-dependent pathway is required for TNF alpha induced apoptosis. Cell. 2003;**5**:61-70. DOI: 10.1016/S0092-8674(03)00757-8

[28] Liu J, Lin A. Role of JNK activation in apoptosis: A double-edged sword. Cell Research. 2005;**15**:36-42. DOI: 10.1038/sj.cr.7290262

Section 2

Structure-activity Studies of Biological Effectiveness in Drug Design and Therapeutic Use

Chapter 4

Indomethacin from Anti-Inflammatory to Anticancer Agent

Shaymaa Emam Kassab

Additional information is available at the end of the chapter

http://dx.doi.org/10.5772/intechopen.79677

Abstract

The chapter "Indomethacin from Anti-inflammatory to Anticancer Agent" covers the recent reports regarding the implication of COX-2/PGE2 in multiple cancer cell proliferation to emphasize the anticancer potential of COX-inhibitors including indomethacin and to reveal that the reduction of PGE2 production interferes with the cancer cell proliferation belongs to multiple cancer cell types. Impressively, indomethacin is involved in antiproliferative and apoptotic actions against cancer cell types via COX-2-independent mechanisms to highlight indomethacin as promising anticancer agent with dual actions to control the cancer cell proliferation. The cardiovascular complications result from diaryl heterocycle sulfonamide/methylsulfone selective COX-2 inhibitors upon reduction in PGE2 and PGI2 production that affects the vascular tone limits the use of Celecoxib as chemopreventive agent against recurrence of colorectal carcinoma cells. Kinetic profile of indomethacin against COX-2 showed obvious difference from that of selective COX-2 inhibitors in which it recovered completely from the enzyme after long time of incubation while COX-2 inhibitors did not recover to impress that this might be implicated in the cardiovascular toxicity of the selective inhibitors. This raised the concern to develop the indomethacin from nonselective COX- to selective COX-2-inhibitors and to assert whether the cardiac complications are from pharmacological class effect or chemical class effect.

Keywords: indomethacin, COX-2-independent mechanism, apoptosis, antiproliferative, kinetic profile

1. Introduction

Indomethacin is indole-3-acetic acid derivative, classified as nonsteriodal anti-inflammatory drug (NSAID). The drug is primarily used for the treatment of painful inflammatory conditions that involves gout and osteoarthritis [1]. The mechanistic role of indomethacin in inhibition of pain has been verified by being nonselective inhibitor to cyclooxygenase-1 (COX-1) and cyclooxygenase-2 (COX-2) isozymes [2]. The enzymatic activity of COX involves bis-oxygenation of arachidonic acid to (prostaglandin G2) PGG2, which then reduced to PGH2 in a peroxidase reaction by the same protein [3]. COX-1 is constitutively expressed in most tissues, to which the production of prostaglandins is attributed to; and COX-2, which is induced by cytokines, mitogens and endotoxins in inflammatory cells, is implicated to the elevated levels of prostaglandins during the inflammation. Prostaglandins are hormone-like mediators involved in the induction of pain, fever and inflammation [2]. The inhibition of indomethacin to the two COX isozymes with minimal selectivity to COX-2 made the drug have serious complications such as gastric ulcers and renal toxicity upon long-term oral administration [4, 5].

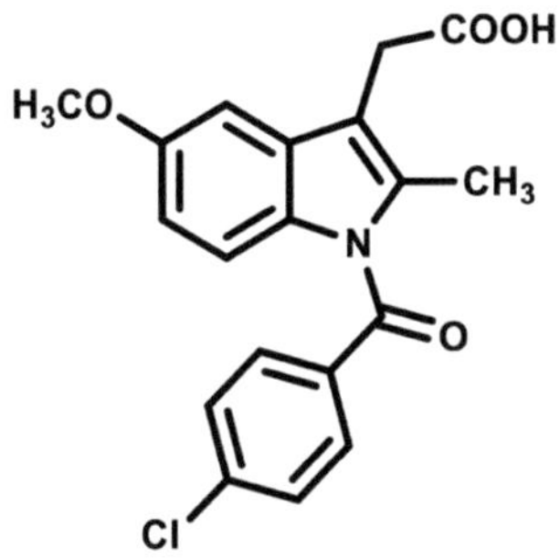

Indomethacin

Indomethacin and the other NSAIDs were found to have significant anticancer activity against wide variety of cancer cell types, *in vitro* and *in vivo* [6–10]. Moreover, epidemiological studies reported that the use of such type of drugs is linked to the reduction of cancer risk [11–13]. Indomethacin performs its anticancer activity in different fashions, inhibits proliferation via induction of apoptic death of tumor cells [6, 9, 10], reduces tumorigenesis by enhancing the immune response [14, 15] and inhibiting the angiogenesis [16, 17] as well.

Interestingly, to mention that the mechanism to which the anticancer activity of NSAIDs including indomethacin attributed is the reduction of PGE2; a type of prostaglandins generated from the bis-oxygenation of arachidonic acid by COX-2. PGE2 contributes to the cell proliferation, cell cycle proliferation and cell cycle progression through various cell signaling mechanisms leads to induction of oncogenic genes and eventually overexpression of proliferative proteins [18–22]. Recently, extensive studies on various cancer cell types including colorectal carcinoma (CRC) justified the efficacy of indomethacin to reduce the levels of antiapoptotic proteins and progressive cell proliferation represented by tumor size by COX-independent mechanisms [23–26].

After emerge and marketing of celecoxib; selective COX-2 inhibitor in December 1998, rofocoxib was released in 1999 worldwide then lumiracoxib and etoricoxib (**Figure 1**) that are marketed in Europe. Those inhibitors are still marketed for the treatment of inflammatory disorders except for rofecoxib and lumiracoxib (the only carboxylic coxib) that were withdrawn due to observation of cardiovascular complications from the recommended daily dose with rofecoxib [27] and observation of liver failure with lumiracoxib [28]. Selective COX-2 inhibitors were launched to treat the individuals who cannot tolerate severe gastrointestinal responses of NSAIDs. A few years later, extensive preclinical and clinical data generated to report the role of COX-2 in tumor growth and/or metastasis [29]. Studies on experimental animals showed that selective COX-2 inhibitors including celecoxib block the formation, growth and metastases of multiple tumor types [30]. Consistently, celecoxib demonstrated dramatic chemopreventive efficacy against colon polyps and reduced the incidence of recurrent adenomas of any type by 45% and of high risk lesions by 66% over a 400 mg dose twice daily for 3 years [31, 32]. One of the complications that should be tackled in the near future for selective COX-2 inhibitors celecoxib in specific is the cardiovascular complications that comes after administration of 400 mg twice daily to be the same as the dose recommended for chemopreventive effect to control the recurrence of CRC [32, 33]. The magnitude of cardiovascular complications of celecoxib limits its use for colon cancer prevention since the development of colon cancer is a slow process, so, the patients with polyps would need to take celecoxib for a long period of time to achieve the target protective effect. Accordingly, a question should be admitted, and should have an evidenced answer: Does the cardiovascular problems of selective COX-2 inhibitors class of anti-inflammatory agent come out of pharmacological class effect or chemical class effect? To my knowledge, we cannot confirm that it is pharmacological class effect and not chemical class effect because the chemical structure of COX-2 inhibitors that share the CVS side effects are Y-shaped diaryl-heterocycle sulfonamide/methylsulfonyl. Thus, it is required to develop new chemical class of selective COX-2 inhibitors help us be provided with verified answer to such important question. The answer of the question would raise the concern to the main reason(s) of CVS complications to tackle and eventually modify the strategy toward generation of selective COX-2 inhibitors with chemopreventive benefits against CRC and other cancer cell types.

Based on the above findings indomethacin, as nonselective COX-inhibitor could be considered strategic lead compound that worth it studying and developing to line it among the chemotherapeutic agents used against cancer to be either prophylactic or therapeutic treatment and/or even adjuvant therapy upon combination with other anticancer agents to

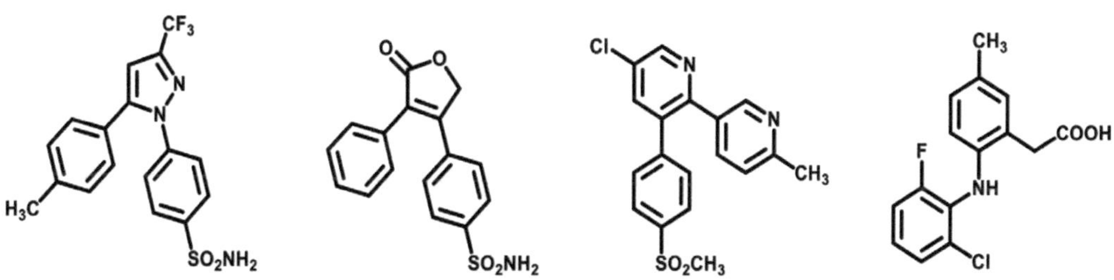

Celecoxib **Rofecoxibe** **Etoricoxib** **Lumiracoxib**

Figure 1. Diarylsulfonamide/methylsulfone selective COX-2 inhibitors.

synergize the chemotherapeutic effect [25]. The subjected insight in this book chapter regarding indomethacin could be easily justified on scientific bases: (1) indomethacin is the most NSAID that is intensively studied as chemopreventive and chemotherapeutic agent against multiple cancer cell types among the other drugs of the same class to show observable results. (2) Indomethacin as a different chemical class when compared to selective COX-2 inhibitors, developing indomethacin-based selective COX-2 inhibitor to excel celecoxib would benefit in asserting whether the cardiovascular system (CVS) problems are originated from chemical class effect. In case, the reason of the cardiovascular system (CVS) complications is attributed to the chemical class effect and indomethacin-based developed structures are devoid of the complications, the patients would be largely benefited from such class of compounds, and it would be chemopreventive agents used for long time without developing cardiovascular system (CVS) complications. (3) Kinetic profile of indomethacin inhibition to COX-2 shows recovery after long time of tight binding to the enzyme [34], and on the other hand, selective COX-2 inhibitors' kinetic profile shows no recovery even after long time of tight binding [35]. This obvious difference between indomethacin and selective COX-2 inhibitors in performing the functionally irreversible inhibition effect to COX-2 has to lead us highlighting indomethacin as promising base to build upon it the developed structures in a way to generate selective COX-2 inhibitors with minimized serious side effects observed with the diaryl heterocycle sulfonamide/methylsulfone class of compounds.

The book chapter covers progressively and in detail some critical topics served in concluding future trends in regard to developing indomethacin to be effective chemopreventive and treatment of various cancer cell types without induction of severe cardiovascular system (CVS) complications: *the implication of COX-2/PGE2 in the anticancer activity of COX-inhibitors, COX-2-independent mechanisms of anticancer activity of indomethacin*, and *significance of indomethacin's anticancer activity over the other NSAIDs and selective COX-2 inhibitors.*

2. Implication of COX-2/PGE2 in anticancer activity of COX-inhibitors

PGE2 implicated in promoting cell proliferation of human esophageal squamous cell carcinoma. The study started with observation of expression and upregulation of c-Myc, an oncogenic transcription factor, and then a link was expected to exist between PGE2 and c-Myc but requires a reliable elucidation. Deeper studies revealed that PGE2 substantially increased the proliferation of cultured esophageal squamous cell carcinoma cells and increased mRNA and protein expression of c-Myc. Moreover, knockdown of c-Myc by RNA interference significantly attenuated PGE2-induced cell proliferation. Furthermore, a mechanistic study described that stability and nuclear accumulation of c-Myc oncogenic protein is attributed PGE2 via phosphorylation on serine 62 that induced by extracellular signal regulated kinase (ERK)-dependent manner and this was confirmed when PGE2 activation of ERK was fully abolished by protein kinase C (PKC) inhibitors. Consistently, PGE2 receptor (EP2) agonist resulted in the same effect on expression of c-Myc as PGE2 and knockdown of EP2 receptor by EP2 small interfering RNA (siRNA) delayed PGE2-induced c-Myc expression to verify the association of PGE2 to c-Myc protein expression in esophageal squamous cancer cell proliferation [18].

It was reported for celecoxib to be effective after Helicobacter Pylori eradication therapy in improving gastric precancerous lesions and stops progression into cancer. The therapeutic effect of celecoxib is explained in the study by measuring the expression and activity of COX-2 for patients with gastric precancerous lesions received celecoxib up to 3 months to be compared with those received placebo for the same period of time. The measurements were determined by immunostaining and PGE2 assay, cell proliferation by Ki-67 immunostaining, apoptosis by TUNEL staining and angiogenesis by microvascular disease (MVD) assay using CD31 staining. The results showed that there was a significant elevation in COX-2 protein expression in gastric precancerous lesions when compared with that resulted from chronic gastritis with consequent increase in cell proliferation and angiogenesis. Patients who were treated with celecoxib showed significant improvement in gastric precancerous lesions (sites of dysplasia) with 84.6% regressed dysplasia, while those treated with placebo showed 60% suggesting that celecoxib was effective on the regression of dysplasia. On the other hand, celecoxib effectively suppressed cell proliferation, induced cell apoptosis and inhibited angiogenesis exhibited by decreased MVD. Interestingly, COX-2 inhibition was accompanied by up-regulation of PPARγ expression that is protective protein with reported antineoplastic effects [36].

Overexpression of COX-2 frequently occurred in head and neck squamous cell carcinoma (HNSCC). COX-2 promotes the release of pro-inflammatory mediator PGE2 which binds to cell surface G-protein coupled receptors EP1–4 to exert its pharmacological effects. Upon studying the biochemical functions of PGE2 and its cell receptors in HNSCC cellular proliferation, it was found that COX-2 and cell receptors EP1, EP2 and EP3 were constitutively expressed in tumoral lesions of HNSCC. An important finding was declared in the study states that small concentration of selective COX-2 inhibitors succeed to suppress PGE2 without inhibition of cell proliferation. However, exogenous addition of EP3-specific agonists with PGE2 induces DNA synthesis in all HNSCC cell lines. Thus, it could be suggested that EP3 receptor subtype of PGE2 should be regarded for future strategies targeting HNSCC prevention [19].

Another study defined a critical mechanism to justify the role of PGE2 in promoting CRC cell division in which prometastatic adaptor protein human enhancer filamentation 1 (HEF1) links between PGE2 and cell cycle machinery in CRC cells. PGE2 induces expression of HEF1 mRNA and protein in CRC. Knockdown of HEF1 suppresses PGE2-induced cell proliferation and cell cycle progression. CRC cells were examined and found that there is 50% elevated levels of HEF1 when compared to normal tissues. Further, HEF1 promotes cell cycle progression of colorectal carcinogenesis via interaction with and activation of cell cycle kinase Aurora A to report that PGE2 is inducer to crucial downstream mediator, HEF1 in colorectal carcinogenesis [20].

Small noncoding RNA, microRNAs (miRNAs) have a key role in stopping the translation and accelerate the degradation of mRNA that regulates the cellular growth and survival through gene suppression. miRNA has a significant contribution in controlling disease progression in pancreatic cancer cells (PaCa). Elevated levels of COX-2 were observed with PGE2 and decrease in miRNA increased the cancer growth and metastases of PaCa. Restoration of miRNA-143 (miR-143) in human PaCa cells reduced COX-2 and inhibited cell proliferation. Mitogen activated kinase (MAPC) was correlated to not detecting miR-143 in some pancreatic cancer cell subtypes to justify the implication of MAPC activation in regulating miR-143 beside COX-2 and PGE2 [21].

$\alpha7$ Nicotinic acetylcholine receptor (nAChR) protein is significantly biosynthesized via cholinergic signaling in nonsmall cell lung cancer (NSCLC) beside COX-2-driven PGE2. The mechanism by which PGE2 promoted NSCLC cell proliferation over α-7 nAChR induction showed the positive effect of PGE2 on $\alpha7$ nAChR expression, promotor activity and cell signaling pathways. The association of the two stimulatory factors to cell growth of NSCLC cells was confirmed upon attenuation of PGE2-induced cell proliferation via $\alpha7$ nAChR siRNA or acetylcholine transferase. Moreover, PGE2 induced $\alpha7$ nAChR production was blocked by EP4 receptor antagonist and EP4 siRNA. Furthermore, it was recorded that blocking c-Jun, critical transcription factor, activated by c-Jun N-terminal kinase (JNK), phosphoinositol 3-kinase (PI3K) and protein kinase A (PKA), led to abolishing the PGE2-induced $\alpha7$ nAChR production and consequent cell growth. It is worthy to mention that activation of JNK, PI3K and PKA resulted from acting of PGE2 on EP4 receptor subtype [22].

Chemopreventive effects of indomethacin was observed for 4-hydroxybutyl(butyl) nitrosamine(OH-BBN)-induced urinary bladder cancers in mice. The study came over conducting three experiments in which the indomethacin was continually administered prior to week 1 or following week 13 OH-BBN dosing for 32 weeks, 1 week after intake of OH-BBN at week 13 for 12 weeks and 30 weeks, and 1 week after intake of OH-BBN at week 13 for 61 weeks, respectively. The chemopreventive effect of indomethacin was observably impressive to show development of palpable bladder masses 3% of animals in case of experiment 1, 77% decrease in palpable masses and 82% decrease in palpable and microscopic masses in case of experiment 2, 26% developed palpable mass under treatment of indomethacin and 66% in control group in case of experiment 3 [26].

3. COX-2-independent mechanisms of anticancer activity of indomethacin

Apoptosis is a programmed cell death induced intrinsically by mitochondrial-mediated or extrinsically by tumor necrosis factor-related apoptosis-inducing ligand (TRAIL)-mediated signals [37]. Caspase activation is generally accompanied by apoptosis that is dependent on mitochondrial mediated or classical extrinsic TRAIL- or death receptor (DR)-mediated signaling [25]. Tse et al. reported the capability of indomethacin to make tumor cells responsive to TRAIL-mediated apoptosis signals through upregulation of TRAIL receptor (DR 5) and down-modulation of survivin, antiapoptic protein [38]. The report provided convincing mechanism to the indomethacin-induced process to overcome TRAIL-resistant melanomas. It is well known that indomethacin enhances mitochondrial oxidative stress and the production of reactive oxygen species (ROS) that modulate mitochondrial-mediated signaling [39]. ROS induces the transcription factor, C/enhancer-binding homologous protein that leads to upregulation of DR 5 on tumor cells. Moreover, ROS has a role in down-modulation of surviving via inhibition of transcription of the known regulator, NF-kB [37]. The report suggests that indomethacin could successfully sensitize TRAIL-resistant melanoma cells.

The ability of indomethacin to work against HCT116 human CRC cells does not express COX was reported using proteomic approach to identify the mechanism by which indomethacin inhibit the CRC growth. The total proteins from indomethacin-treated and untreated cancer cells were separated by immobilized pH gradient-based two-dimensional gel electrophoresis. The different proteins produced throughout the test were identified by peptide mass fingerprint (PMF) based on matrix-assisted laser desorption/ionization time of flight mass spectrometry. The results revealed that indomethacin induced HCT116 apoptosis and inhibited cell growth by downregulation Wnt1-inducible signaling pathway protein 1, Bcl-2-related protein A1 and mitogen-activated protein kinase [24].

c-AMP activates PKA in and c-AMP-response element binding (CREB) protein in melanogenesis. CREB plays an important role in binding to the promotor of the microphthalmia-associated transcription factor (Mitf) gene and consequently activates Mitf gene transcription [40, 41]. Thus, Mitf has a crucial role in transcription of melanogenic genes and activates melanogenic gene transcription of tyrosinase as well. Indomethacin was studied to investigate the effect on melanogenesis in B16F1 melanoma cells. The study resulted in indomethacin inhibited α-melanocyte stimulating hormone that enhances melanin synthesis in melanoma cells., suppressed tyrosinase and Mitf protein levels, reduced tyrosinase promoter activity, lowered mRNA of melanogenic genes, including Mitf gene [23].

AMP-protein kinase (AMPK) is a key factor of master regulation of cellular energy homeostasis [42]. When AMPK is activated, it induces block of cell cycle and apoptotic cell death in different types of cancer cells including gliomas, the primary tumors of central nervous system [43–47]. The apoptotic death and inhibition of growth of cancer cell actions of AMPK are mediated by one of the signaling pathway in which mammalian target of rapamycin (mTOR) is inhibited. It is worthy to note that mTOR is a catalytic core for formation of two definite complexes, mTOR complex 1 (mTORC1) and 2 (mTORC2) and both are sensitive targets to rapamycin, allosteric inhibitor of the complexes [48]. mTORC1 has a supporting role in protein synthesis and cell proliferation. mTOR performs its biological functions by phosphorylating ribosomal p70S6 kinase and translational repressor 4E-BP1 [48]. AMPK phosphorylates raptor and/or tuberous sclerosis complex-mediated inhibition of mTOR stimulator Ras homolog enriched in brain (RHEB) [49]. Beside the role of mTORC1 in cell proliferation, it causes major and observable negative regulation to intracellular degradation of unnecessary and dysfunctional cellular components through lysosomal machinery which is a kind of cytotoxic mechanism [50]. Indomethacin was reported as growth inhibitor to CRC cells by mTOR inhibition [51]. For the glioma cells U251, indomethacin showed superior *in vitro* antiglioma action and restriction to cell proliferation to the other COX-inhibitors when tested against the same cancer cells. The antiproliferative and proapoptotic actions of indomethacin against U251 was evidenced by G2M cell cycle arrest P21 associated with caspase-3/9 activation, DNA fragmentation that were displayed by indomethacin-treated glioma cells [52]. Also, indomethacin stimulates AMPK phosphorylation in glioma cells and the implication of this pathway in antiglioma effect of indomethacin was confirmed by knockdown of AMPK via RNA interference to alter the AMPK activity and antiglioma actions of indomethacin. Generally, AMPK seemed not sufficient antiproliferative pathway to restrict glioma cell proliferation. Therefore, it is expected that treating glioma cells with indomethacin had a synergistic effect came from its AMPK-dependent and -independent pathways in inhibiting the cancer cell growth and proliferation of gliomas.

4. Significance of indomethacin and its developed structures' anticancer activity over the other NSAIDs and selective COX-2 inhibitors

According to the literature scan had been done on indomethacin as nonselective COX-inhibitor and antiproliferative agent, it could be observed that indomethacin is the most NSAID that attracted the interest of researchers to study, investigate, identify more about the definite mechanisms and cellular signaling pathways involved in the antiproliferative and apoptotic effects of indomethacin. This might be attributed to two apparent points: one is the observable inhibition of cell growth, reduction of tumor size and implication in the programmed cell death of multiple tumor cell types including glioma and glioblastomas that require lipophilicity for cell penetration. The second is that indomethacin exhibited its anticancer activity against wide variety of cancer cell types by COX-2/PGE2-dependent and -independent mechanisms. This adds great advantage to indomethacin over the other nonselective COX-inhibitors because in that way, indomethacin has dual actions by which it could exert its cytotoxic activity effectively.

Regarding the selective COX-2 inhibitors, the prophylactic actions of celecoxib against recurrence of colon polyps is defined by researchers as dramatic to indicate the capability of celecoxib and other COX-2 inhibitors to block the cancer cell growth and metastases as well. One serious complication that is developed upon long-term therapy of celecoxib that limits its use as chemopreventive therapy for CRC is the cardiovascular toxicity that results from critical reduction in PGE2 and prostacyclin (PGI2) production. Those types of prostaglandins are COX2-dependent product responsible for regulating vascular tone and atherosclerosis [53]. The problem is absolutely the same as all the selective COX-2 inhibitors since they share the same pharmacological action in which production of prostaglandins is significantly diminished.

Some differential points related to the kinetic profile of both indomethacin [34] and selective COX-2 inhibitors [35] were worth it stopping at to help us draw a future plan to develop indomethacin's chemical structure in a way to enhance COX-2 inhibition activity like selective COX-2 inhibitors and be devoid of cardiovascular complications as well. Nonselective inhibitors including indomethacin perform its inhibition action against the enzyme through 2-step inhibition mechanism involving slow and time-dependent step due to tight reversible binding to the enzyme to be considered as functionally irreversible. But selective COX-2 inhibitors inhibit the enzyme through 3-step inhibition mechanism involving time-dependent step that represents the tightly bound complex of inhibited enzyme. The observation that should be highlighted for both types of COX-inhibitors while monitoring the kinetic model of inhibition mechanism is that indomethacin carboxylic acid is not essential for the tight binding and time-dependent step of enzyme inhibition because the esterified counterpart did not abolish this step or even reduce the tightness of binding to human COX-2 and the formation of the complex maintained functionally irreversible [54, 55]. Further, indomethacin recovered intact after prolonged time of incubation with the enzyme, this suggests that enzyme inhibition came over conformational change not covalent bond formation [34]. On the other hand, DuP 697, selective COX-2 inhibitor showed the same time-dependent step that was responsible for drug's selective inhibition of human COX-2 but impressively the inhibitor did not show successful recovery even upon dialysis but the inhibitor is freed to inhibit another enzyme under the effect of denaturation to confirm that the tight binding of inhibitor to the enzyme was not based on formation of covalent bond [35].

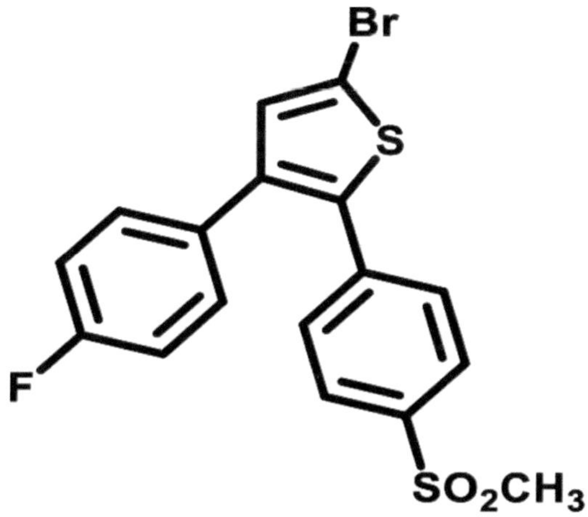

DuP 697

The detrimental differences in regard to the kinetic profile of indomethacin, nonselective COX-inhibitor and DuP 697, selective COX-2 inhibitor for inhibition of COX-2 raised my concern with that emerge of developed selective COX-2 inhibitors based on indomethacin would definitely help us answer two important questions:

i. *Is the cardiovascular toxicity of selective COX-2 inhibitors pharmacological class effect of chemical class effect?* The change of chemical class of selective COX-2 inhibitors from the traditional diaryl heterocycle sulfonamide/methylsulfone to indomethacin-based structures and identifying the kinetic profile of the new class of selective inhibitors would provide a strong evidence on the real reasons of cardiovascular problems after administration of selective COX-2 inhibitors to discover whether it lies behind the kinetic mode of enzyme inhibition which depends on the chemical structure or it lies behind the selective action of the drug against COX-2. In case of similar kinetic profile for the generated new inhibitors to the traditional class and no recovery to the inhibitor is shown, so, it will imply that it is a general feature to the selective inhibitors whatever is the chemical structure. It could be drawn that the inability of selective inhibitors to get recovered from COX-2 enzyme might be a significant reason to the CVS complications of the inhibitors. In case, the new structures saved the kinetic profile of the original lead compound, indomethacin, so, it would be worth it monitoring the development of CVS problems after long-term administration of the newly developed indomethacin-based compounds. There are two reports based on epidemiological studies stated clearly that prolonged use of NSAIDs is associated by small increase in CVS risk [56, 57]. This attracted our attention to comment on that this happens though NSAIDs inhibit COX-2 with the same efficacy as selective

COX-2 inhibitors. Thus, it is suggested that chemical structure and/or binding mode most likely play a significant role in determining the kinetic mode of enzyme inhibition. But, we are still in serious need to an evidence results from experimental studies to assertively answer the above question.

ii. *Would the anticancer activity of indomethacin be enhanced with the new indomethacin-based compounds?* Improvement of the selective inhibition of COX-2 in comparison to indomethacin is supposed to potentiate the antiproliferative and apoptotic activities upon enhanced diminishing to COX-2/PGE2, combining this important signaling pathway with the COX-2-independent mechanisms of anticancer activities that previously described in this book chapter for indomethacin in Section 2 "COX-2-independent mechanisms of anticancer activity of indomethacin".

Several attempts for generation of indomethacin-based analogs of selective COX-2 inhibition activity [58–60], but the publication that I had to put it in focus in this regard is that described the design and synthesis of indomethacin-based analogs of potentially selective COX-2 inhibition activity and observed diminishing to PGE2 [61]. The successful generation of developed indomethacin structures with selective COX-2 inhibition activity was iteratively reported in the literature but picking this publication to comment on among the others was based on the obvious selectivity index of the generated analogs that excelled celecoxib, dramatic lowering to plasma levels of PGE2 when compared to indomethacin, the innovative perspective upon

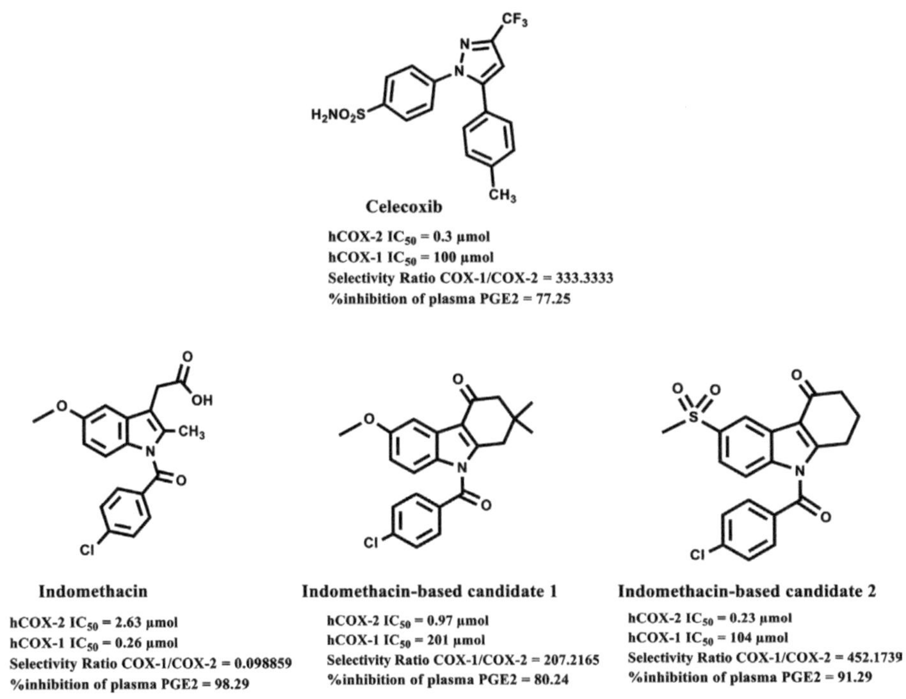

Figure 2. Biological data of the new indomethacin-based selective COX-2 inhibitors 1 and 2 in comparison with indomethacin and celecoxib.

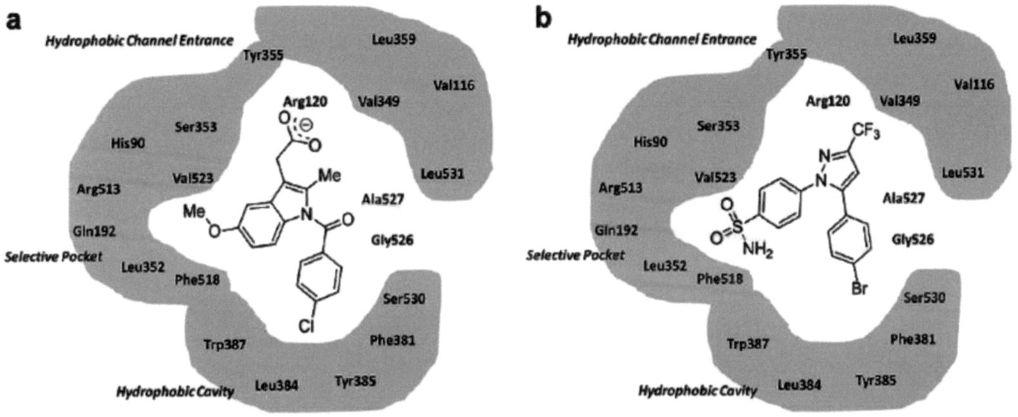

Figure 3. Schematic representation of SC-558 (COX-2 selective inhibitor) binding to COX-2 (a) and indomethacin (nonselective inhibitor) (b).

which the design and modification of the analogs are designed, and above all of this the biological profiling through multiple *in vitro* and *in vivo* tests that done for the analogs to impress the discovery of interesting tetrahydrocarbazole candidates. Accordingly, the newly selective COX-2 inhibitors worth it promoting to study how far it is implicated in CVS toxicity upon long-term therapy against either cancer or inflammatory diseases.

The new tetrahydrocarbazole selective COX-2 inhibitors **(1)** and **(2)** (**Figure 2**) generated were based on enlarging the size of indomethacin indole ring to occupy the wider catalytic pocket of COX-2 than COX-2 by 25% [62] and reducing the opportunity of the ring-extended candidates to interact with COX-1 to raise the selectivity. Introduction of methyl sulfonyl group to replace methoxy group of indomethacin at position 6 to enhance the interaction of the designed inhibitor **(2)** (**Figure 3**) with the polar side pocket of COX-2 (selective pocket) that is critical for COX-2 inhibition activity [63]. Deletion of carboxylic acid from the new candidates **(1)** and **(2)** reduce the possibility of the inhibitor to interact with COX-1 via formation of salt bridge with Arg120 amino acid (**Figure 3**) [64] that is critical for conformational change and inhibition of the isoenzyme. Impressively, the biological results throughout *in vitro* testing represented by enzymatic assays against human COX-1 (hCOX-1) and hCOX-2 and *in vivo* testing represented by % inhibition of plasma PGE2 and others revealed the successful verification of the proposed hypothesis suggested to enhance the COX-2 inhibition selectivity. Methoxy derivative **(1)** (**Figure 2**) gave selectivity index against COX-2 (207.2165) to excel both that of indomethacin (0.98859) and celecoxib (333.3333) standard drugs. For the methylsulfone derivative **(2)** (**Figure 2**), it excelled the standard materials at much higher value (452.1739). Moreover, the diminishing of plasma levels of PGE2 was very observable in comparison to indomethacin (98.29%) and celecoxib (77.25%) (**Figure 2**). Thus, kinetic profile of the enzyme inhibition of the new candidate **(2)** in the near future would answer the questions described in this section on the book and eventually be able to judge on the chemopreventive of the new selective COX-2 inhibitor and antiproliferative activity as well.

5. Conclusions

Generation of indomethacin-based analogs to indomethacin aiming at enhancing the selective COX-2 inhibition would definitely help us answer an important question concerning the real reason of cardiovascular toxicity of selective COX-2 inhibitors, whether it is pharmacological class effect or chemical class effect. Moreover, enhancing the selectivity of indomethacin against COX-2 among the other NSAIDs providing a candidate privileged with potential anti-inflammatory activity devoid of gastrointestinal side effects and what is more important is obtaining newly developed structure carries effective antiproliferative and apoptotic activity standing for the dual actions reported for indomethacin as a lead compound based on that it performs its anticancer activity by both COX-2-dependent and COX-2-independent mechanisms. Further, the CVS toxicity is expected to be minimized upon enhancing the selective COX-2 inhibition of indomethacin due to observation that there might be a difference in the kinetic mode of enzyme inhibition between diaryl heterocycle sulfonamide/methylsulfone chemical class of selective COX-2 inhibitors and the new indomethacin-based chemical class of compounds that may permit successful recovery of the new inhibitors from the enzyme after long incubation period.

Nomenclature

NSAID	nonsteroidal anti-inflammatory drug
COX	cyclooxygenase
PG	prostaglandin
CRC	colorectal carcinoma
CVS	cardiovascular
ERK	extracellular signal regulated kinase
PKC	protein kinase C
siRNA	small interfering RNA
MVD	microvascular d
HNSCC	head and neck small cell carcinoma
HEF1	human enhancer filamentation 1
miRNA	microRNA
MAPC	mitogen activated kinase
NSCLC	nonsmall cell lung cancer
JNK	c-Jun N-terminal kinase

PI3K	phosphoinositol 3-kinase
PKA	protein kinase A
OH-BBN	4-hydroxybutyl(butyl)nitrosamine
TRAIL	tumor necrosis factor-related apoptosis-inducing ligand
DR	death receptor
ROS	reactive oxygen species
PMF	protein mass fingerprint
CREB	c-AMP-response element binding
AMPK	adenosine monophosphate kinase
mTOR	mammalian target of rapamycin
RHEB	Ras homolog enriched in brain

Author details

Shaymaa Emam Kassab

Address all correspondence to: shaymaa.kassab@pharm.dmu.edu.eg

Faulty of Pharmacy, Pharmaceutical Chemistry Department, Damanhour University, Damanhour, El-Buhaira, Egypt

References

[1] Suleyman H, Albayrak A, Bilici M, Cadirci E, Halici Z. Different mechanisms in formation and prevention of indomethacin-induced gastric ulcers. Inflammation. 2010;**33**:224-234

[2] Guo YC, Chang CM, Hsu WL, Chiu SJ, Tsai YT, Chou YH, Hou MF, Wang JY, Lee MH, Tsai KL, Chang WC. Indomethacin inhibits cancer cell migration via attenuation of cellular calcium mobilization. Molecules (Basel, Switzerland). 2013;**18**:6584-6596

[3] Smith WL, Urade Y, Jakobsson PJ. Enzymes of the cyclooxygenase pathways of prostanoid biosynthesis. Chemical Reviews. 2011;**111**:5821-5865

[4] Zarghi A, Arfaei S. Selective COX-2 inhibitors: A review of their structure-activity relationships. Iranian Journal of Pharmaceutical research: IJPR. 2011;**10**:655-683

[5] Peesa JP, Yalavarthi PR, Rasheed A, Mandava VBR. A perspective review on role of novel NSAID prodrugs in the management of acute inflammation. Journal of Acute Disease. 2016;**5**:364-381

[6] Brunelli C, Amici C, Angelini M, Fracassi C, Belardo G, Santoro MG. The non-steroidal anti-inflammatory drug indomethacin activates the eIF2alpha kinase PKR, causing a translational block in human colorectal cancer cells. The Biochemical Journal. 2012; **443**:379-386

[7] Elder DJ, Hague A, Hicks DJ, Paraskeva C. Differential growth inhibition by the aspirin metabolite salicylate in human colorectal tumor cell lines: Enhanced apoptosis in carcinoma and in vitro-transformed adenoma relative to adenoma relative to adenoma cell lines. Cancer Research. 1996;**56**:2273-2276

[8] Elder DJ, Halton DE, Hague A, Paraskeva C. Induction of apoptotic cell death in human colorectal carcinoma cell lines by a cyclooxygenase-2 (COX-2)-selective nonsteroidal anti-inflammatory drug: Independence from COX-2 protein expression. Clinical Cancer Research: An Official Journal of the American Association for Cancer Research. 1997; **3**:1679-1683

[9] Eli Y, Przedecki F, Levin G, Kariv NA, Raz A. Comparative effects of indomethacin on cell proliferation and cell cycle progression in tumor cells grown in vitro and in vivo. Biochemical Pharmacology. 2001;**61**:565-571

[10] Hojka-Osinska A, Ziolo E, Rapak A. Combined treatment with fenretinide and indomethacin induces AIF-mediated, non-classical cell death in human acute T-cell leukemia Jurkat cells. Biochemical and Biophysical Research Communications. 2012;**419**:590-595

[11] Bosetti C, Rosato V, Gallus S, Cuzick J, La Vecchia C. Aspirin and cancer risk: A quantitative review to. Annals of Oncology: Official Journal of the European Society for Medical Oncology. 2011;**23**(2012):1403-1415

[12] Johannesdottir SA, Chang ET, Mehnert F, Schmidt M, Olesen AB, Sorensen HT. Nonsteroidal anti-inflammatory drugs and the risk of skin cancer: A population-based case-control study. Cancer. 2012;**118**:4768-4776

[13] Takkouche B, Regueira-Mendez C, Etminan M. Breast cancer and use of nonsteroidal anti-inflammatory drugs: A meta-analysis. Journal of the National Cancer Institute. 2008; **100**:1439-1447

[14] Jukic MK, Luetic AT, Skudar-Lukinovic V, Andreis I. The antimetastatic effect of macrophages restored by indomethacin: Concomitant tumor immunity model. Collegium Antropologicum. 2010;**34**:899-904

[15] Morecki S, Yacovlev E, Gelfand Y, Trembovler V, Shohami E, Slavin S. Induction of antitumor immunity by indomethacin. Cancer Immunology, Immunotherapy. 2000;**48**:613-620

[16] Bigda J, Mysliwski A. Indomethacin inhibits kidney metastasis in bomirski melanoma-bearing hamsters, and modulates natural killer cytotoxic activity of tumor hosts in vivo and in vitro. Anticancer Research. 1998;**18**:3549-3554

[17] Levin G, Kariv N, Khomiak E, Raz A. Indomethacin inhibits the accumulation of tumor cells in mouse lungs and subsequent growth of lung metastases. Chemotherapy. 2000; **46**:429-437

[18] Le Y, Kei WWK, Jie LZ, Tao LH, Chun WY, Hin CC. Prostaglandin E2 promotes cell proliferation via protein kinase C/extracellular signal regulated kinase pathway-dependent induction of c-Myc expression in human esophageal squamous cell carcinoma cells. International Journal of Cancer. 2009;**125**:2540-2546

[19] Abrahao AC, Castilho RM, Squarize CH, Molinolo AA, Santos-Pinto DD Jr, Gutkind JS. A role for COX2-derived PGE2 and PGE2-receptor subtypes in head and neck squamous carcinoma cell proliferation. Oral Oncology. 2010;**46**:880-887

[20] Xia D, Holla VR, Wang D, Menter DG, DuBois RN. HEF1 is a crucial mediator of the proliferative effects of prostaglandin E(2) on colon cancer cells. Cancer Research. 2010;**70**:824-831

[21] Pham H, Ekaterina Rodriguez C, Donald GW, Hertzer KM, Jung XS, Chang H-H, Moro A, Reber HA, Hines OJ, Eibl G. miR-143 decreases COX-2 mRNA stability and expression in pancreatic cancer cells. Biochemical and Biophysical Research Communications. 2013;**439**:6-11

[22] Xiao Rong Z, Yu F, Ritzenthaler JD, Wen Jing Z, Ke W, Qing Hua Z, Jesse R. Novel link between prostaglandin E2 (PGE2) and cholinergic signaling in lung cancer: The role of c-Jun in PGE2-induced $\alpha7$ nicotinic acetylcholine receptor expression and tumor cell proliferation. Thoracic Cancer. 2015;**6**:488-500

[23] Sato K, Takei M, Iyota R, Muraoka Y, Nagashima M, Yoshimura Y. Indomethacin inhibits melanogenesis via down-regulation of Mitf mRNA transcription. Bioscience, Biotechnology, and Biochemistry. 2017;**81**:2307-2313

[24] Cheng YL, Zhang GY, Li C, Lin J. Screening for novel protein targets of indomethacin in HCT116 human colon cancer cells using proteomics. Oncology Letters. 2013;**6**:1222-1228

[25] Somasundaram R, Herlyn M. Indomethacin to the rescue of TRAIL-resistant melanomas. The Journal of Investigative Dermatology. 2014;**134**:1198-1199

[26] Lubet RA, Huebner K, Fong LY, Altieri DC, Steele VE, Kopelovich L, Kavanaugh C, Juliana MM, Soong SJ, Grubbs CJ. 4-Hydroxybutyl(butyl)nitrosamine-induced urinary bladder cancers in mice: Characterization of FHIT and survivin expression and chemopreventive effects of indomethacin. Carcinogenesis. 2005;**26**:571-578

[27] Bresalier RS, Sandler RS, Quan H, Bolognese JA, Oxenius B, Horgan K, Lines C, Riddell R, Morton D, Lanas A, Konstam MA, Baron JA. Cardiovascular events associated with rofecoxib in a colorectal adenoma chemoprevention trial. The New England Journal of Medicine. 2005;**352**:1092-1102

[28] Shi S, Klotz U. Clinical use and pharmacological properties of selective COX-2 inhibitors. European Journal of Clinical Pharmacology. 2008;**64**:233-252

[29] Thun MJ, Henley SJ, Patrono C. Nonsteroidal anti-inflammatory drugs as anticancer agents: Mechanistic, pharmacologic, and clinical issues. Journal of the National Cancer Institute. 2002;**94**:252-266

[30] Gupta RA, Dubois RN. Colorectal cancer prevention and treatment by inhibition of cyclooxygenase-2. Nature Reviews. Cancer. 2001;**1**:11-21

[31] Arber N, Eagle CJ, Spicak J, Racz I, Dite P, Hajer J, Zavoral M, Lechuga MJ, Gerletti P, Tang J, Rosenstein RB, Macdonald K, Bhadra P, Fowler R, Wittes J, Zauber AG, Solomon SD, Levin B. Celecoxib for the prevention of colorectal adenomatous polyps. The New England Journal of Medicine. 2006;**355**:885-895

[32] Bertagnolli MM, Eagle CJ, Zauber AG, Redston M, Solomon SD, Kim K, Tang J, Rosenstein RB, Wittes J, Corle D, Hess TM, Woloj GM, Boisserie F, Anderson WF, Viner JL, Bagheri D, Burn J, Chung DC, Dewar T, Foley TR, Hoffman N, Macrae F, Pruitt RE, Saltzman JR, Salzberg B, Sylwestrowicz T, Gordon GB, Hawk ET. Celecoxib for the prevention of sporadic colorectal adenomas. The New England Journal of Medicine. 2006;**355**: 873-884

[33] Psaty BM, Potter JD. Risks and benefits of celecoxib to prevent recurrent adenomas. The New England Journal of Medicine. 2006;**355**:950-952

[34] Kulmacz RJ, Lands WE. Stoichiometry and kinetics of the interaction of prostaglandin H synthase with anti-inflammatory agents. The Journal of Biological Chemistry. 1985;**260**:12572-12578

[35] Copeland RA, Williams JM, Giannaras J, Nurnberg S, Covington M, Pinto D, Pick S, Trzaskos JM. Mechanism of selective inhibition of the inducible isoform of prostaglandin G/H synthase. Proceedings of the National Academy of Sciences of the United States of America. 1994;**91**:11202-11206

[36] Zhang L-J, Wang S-Y, Huo X-H, Zhu Z-L, Chu J-K, Ma J-C, Cui D-S, Gu P, Zhao Z-R, Wang M-W, Yu J. Anti-helicobacter pylori therapy followed by celecoxib on progression of gastric precancerous lesions. World Journal of Gastroenterology: WJG. 2009;**15**:2731-2738

[37] Hersey P, Zhang XD. How melanoma cells evade trail-induced apoptosis. Nature Reviews. Cancer. 2001;**1**:142-150

[38] Tse AK, Cao HH, Cheng CY, Kwan HY, Yu H, Fong WF, Yu ZL. Indomethacin sensitizes TRAIL-resistant melanoma cells to TRAIL-induced apoptosis through ROS-mediated upregulation of death receptor 5 and downregulation of survivin. The Journal of Investigative Dermatology. 2014;**134**:1397-1407

[39] Maity P, Bindu S, Dey S, Goyal M, Alam A, Pal C, Mitra K, Bandyopadhyay U. Indomethacin, a non-steroidal anti-inflammatory drug, develops gastropathy by inducing reactive oxygen species-mediated mitochondrial pathology and associated apoptosis in gastric mucosa: A novel role of mitochondrial aconitase oxidation. The Journal of Biological Chemistry. 2009;**284**:3058-3068

[40] Steingrimsson E, Copeland NG, Jenkins NA. Melanocytes and the microphthalmia transcription factor network. Annual Review of Genetics. 2004;**38**:365-411

[41] Bertolotto C, Abbe P, Hemesath TJ, Bille K, Fisher DE, Ortonne JP, Ballotti R. Microphthalmia gene product as a signal transducer in cAMP-induced differentiation of melanocytes. The Journal of Cell Biology. 1998;**142**:827-835

[42] Hardie DG, Ashford ML. AMPK: Regulating energy balance at the cellular and whole body levels. Physiology (Bethesda, Md.). 2014;**29**:99-107

[43] Campas C, Lopez JM, Santidrian AF, Barragan M, Bellosillo B, Colomer D, Gil J. Acadesine activates AMPK and induces apoptosis in B-cell chronic lymphocytic leukemia cells but not in T lymphocytes. Blood. 2003;**101**:3674-3680

[44] Chen MB, Zhang Y, Wei MX, Shen W, Wu XY, Yao C, Lu PH. Activation of AMP-activated protein kinase (AMPK) mediates plumbagin-induced apoptosis and growth inhibition in cultured human colon cancer cells. Cellular Signalling. 2013;**25**:1993-2002

[45] Isakovic A, Harhaji L, Stevanovic D, Markovic Z, Sumarac-Dumanovic M, Starcevic V, Micic D, Trajkovic V. Dual antiglioma action of metformin: Cell cycle arrest and mitochondria-dependent apoptosis. Cellular and Molecular Life Sciences: CMLS. 2007; **64**:1290-1302

[46] Nieminen AI, Eskelinen VM, Haikala HM, Tervonen TA, Yan Y, Partanen JI, Klefstrom J. Myc-induced AMPK-phospho p53 pathway activates Bak to sensitize mitochondrial apoptosis. Proceedings of the National Academy of Sciences of the United States of America. 2013;**110**:E1839-E1848

[47] Wang B, Wang XB, Chen LY, Huang L, Dong RZ. Belinostat-induced apoptosis and growth inhibition in pancreatic cancer cells involve activation of TAK1-AMPK signaling axis. Biochemical and Biophysical Research Communications. 2013;**437**:1-6

[48] Morita M, Gravel SP, Hulea L, Larsson O, Pollak M, St-Pierre J, Topisirovic I. mTOR coordinates protein synthesis, mitochondrial activity and proliferation. Cell Cycle (Georgetown, Texas). 2015;**14**:473-480

[49] Inoki K, Kim J, Guan KL. AMPK and mTOR in cellular energy homeostasis and drug targets. Annual Review of Pharmacology and Toxicology. 2012;**52**:381-400

[50] Yang Z, Klionsky DJ. Mammalian autophagy: Core molecular machinery and signaling regulation. Current Opinion in Cell Biology. 2010;**22**:124-131

[51] Zhang YJ, Bao YJ, Dai Q, Yang WY, Cheng P, Zhu LM, Wang BJ, Jiang FH. mTOR signaling is involved in indomethacin and nimesulide suppression of colorectal cancer cell growth via a COX-2 independent pathway. Annals of Surgical Oncology. 2011;**18**:580-588

[52] Pantovic A, Bosnjak M, Arsikin K, Kosic M, Mandic M, Ristic B, Tosic J, Grujicic D, Isakovic A, Micic N, Trajkovic V, Harhaji-Trajkovic L. In vitro antiglioma action of indomethacin is mediated via AMP-activated protein kinase/mTOR complex 1 signalling pathway. The International Journal of Biochemistry & Cell Biology. 2017;**83**:84-96

[53] Moncada S, Higgs EA, Vane JR. Human arterial and venous tissues generate prostacyclin (prostaglandin x), a potent inhibitor of platelet aggregation. Lancet (London, England). 1977;**1**:18-20

[54] Greig GM, Francis DA, Falgueyret JP, Ouellet M, Percival MD, Roy P, Bayly C, Mancini JA, O'Neill GP. The interaction of arginine 106 of human prostaglandin G/H synthase-2 with inhibitors is not a universal component of inhibition mediated by nonsteroidal anti-inflammatory drugs. Molecular Pharmacology. 1997;**52**:829-838

[55] Kalgutkar AS, Crews BC, Rowlinson SW, Marnett AB, Kozak KR, Remmel RP, Marnett LJ. Biochemically based design of cyclooxygenase-2 (COX-2) inhibitors: Facile conversion of nonsteroidal antiinflammatory drugs to potent and highly selective COX-2 inhibitors. Proceedings of the National Academy of Sciences of the United States of America. 2000;**97**:925-930

[56] Hippisley-Cox J, Coupland C. Risk of myocardial infarction in patients taking cyclooxygenase-2 inhibitors or conventional non-steroidal anti-inflammatory drugs: Population based nested case-control analysis. BMJ (Clinical research ed.). 2005;**330**:1366

[57] Garcia Rodriguez LA, Gonzalez-Perez A. Long-term use of non-steroidal anti-inflammatory drugs and the risk of myocardial infarction in the general population. BMC Medicine. 2005;**3**:17

[58] Blobaum AL, Uddin MJ, Felts AS, Crews BC, Rouzer CA, Marnett LJ. The 2′-Trifluoromethyl analogue of indomethacin is a potent and selective COX-2 inhibitor. ACS Medicinal Chemistry Letters. 2013;**4**:486-490

[59] Lau CK, Black WC, Belley M, Chan C, Charleson S, Denis D, Gauthier JY, Gordon R, Guay D, Hamel P, Kargman S, Leblanc Y, Mancini J, Ouellet M, Percival D, Prasit P, Roy P, Skorey K, Tagari P, Vickers P, Wong E. From indomethacin to a selective COX-2 inhibitor. Development of indolalkanoic acids as potent and selective cyclooxygenase-2 inhibitors. Advances in Experimental Medicine and Biology. 1997;**407**:73-78

[60] Estevao MS, Carvalho LC, Freitas M, Gomes A, Viegas A, Manso J, Erhardt S, Fernandes E, Cabrita EJ, Marques MM. Indole based cyclooxygenase inhibitors: Synthesis, biological evaluation, docking and NMR screening. European Journal of Medicinal Chemistry. 2012;**54**:823-833

[61] Kassab SE, Khedr MA, Ali HI, Abdalla MM. Discovery of new indomethacin-based analogs with potentially selective cyclooxygenase-2 inhibition and observed diminishing to PGE2 activities. European Journal of Medicinal Chemistry. 2017;**141**:306-321

[62] Luong C, Miller A, Barnett J, Chow J, Ramesha C, Browner MF. Flexibility of the NSAID binding site in the structure of human cyclooxygenase-2. Nature Structural Biology. 1996; **3**:927-933

[63] Dwivedi AK, Gurjar V, Kumar S, Singh N. Molecular basis for nonspecificity of nonsteroidal anti-inflammatory drugs (NSAIDs). Drug Discovery Today. 2015;**20**:863-873

[64] Estevão MS, Carvalho LCR, Freitas M, Gomes A, Viegas A, Manso J, Erhardt S, Fernandes E, Cabrita EJ, Marques MMB. Indole based cyclooxygenase inhibitors: Synthesis, biological evaluation, docking and NMR screening. European Journal of Medicinal Chemistry. 2012;**54**:823-833

Chapter 5

1,4-Benzodiazepines and New Derivatives: Description, Analysis, and Organic Synthesis

Elisabet Batlle, Enric Lizano, Miquel Viñas and
Maria Dolors Pujol

Additional information is available at the end of the chapter

http://dx.doi.org/10.5772/intechopen.79879

Abstract

Benzodiazepines are widely used drugs for several indications. This study provides, on the other hand, a global vision of the family starting for their fortuitous discovery, the synthesis of their derivatives, their mechanism of action widely known nowadays, the actual classification according to the chemical structure and pharmacokinetic properties, and their uses and indications, the traditional and the new ones. On the other hand,the study is focused in the mainly problems of benzodiazepines, depedence, and tolerance, many times led by a misuse of the patient, wrong prescriptions, or extended treatments. A withdrawal program is proposed that includes the important factors or criteria to success, with a slow and gradual reduction of these drugs, avoiding relapse or severe adverse effects. New lines of research related to benzodiazepines are taken into account, which not only include the new therapeutic uses but also the adverse effects in short and long term. They are also analyzed the new discoveries concerning the nonbenzodiazepine drugs due to the close relation they have with benzodiazepines.

Keywords: benzodiazepines, withdrawal program, nonbenzodiazepine drugs, biological activities, side effects

1. Discovery and history

Many of the drugs that had represented a great advance in many therapeutic approaches were not a result of a rational design but of a consequence of casual observations, fortuitous discoveries, or serendipity. Way back then, a rational design did not guarantee the exit because the knowledge of the biological systems was not clear or complete. That happened in the beginning of the past century, and many of the drugs used nowadays come from this type of discovery, from the curiosity of many investigators that decided to study the reason why they were not achieving their goals.

Discovery starts with chemist Leo Sternbach and his research group, working in the Hoffmann-La Roche laboratories in Nutley, New Jersey. They were trying to find new tranquilizers, but due to the limited knowledge of the processes occurring in the brain, they were taking an empirical approach: to search for a new class of drugs purely guided by modifications in the known chemical synthesis [1]. In 1957, they serendipitously identified the first benzodiazepine (BZD), *chlordiazepoxide*, while they were studying the activity of *quinazoline oxide*. They saw that the compound obtained was not a quinazoline-N^3-oxide but a benzodiazepine-N^4-oxide. With a posterior investigation, Sternbach himself managed to explain what happened [2].

By 1960, Hoffmann-La Roche introduced the *chlordiazepoxide* in clinical treatment under the brand name Librium®, and it pursued molecular modifications to improve its activity. By the time of its introduction, it was felt that an explanation of the BZDs mechanism of action might be really helpful to understand the basis of anxiety. *Diazepam* (Valium®) followed in 1963, which was considered for a long time as head of the family.

An important improvement was their lack of respiratory depression, a safety concern they had with barbiturates [3].

Medical professionals accepted benzodiazepines enthusiastically at first, increasing their popularity and patient demand. BZDs were prescribed frequently and often long term for various conditions. Soon they became the pharmacological family *par excellence* in the treatment of anxiety disorders and so initiating "the benzodiazepine saga" [4].

It took 15 years for the researchers to associate benzodiazepines and their effect with their high-affinity receptor complex as a mechanism of action. They did it in 1977, and it was the major turning point in the research [2].

1.1. Benzodiazepines (BZDs)

Benzodiazepines are a structural class of compounds that are used as hypnotics, anxiolytics, anticonvulsants, and muscle relaxants. Their core chemical structure is formed by the fusion of a benzene ring and a diazepine ring (**Figure 1**). Different compounds have different side groups attached to this central structure in position 1, 2, 5, or 7. The different side groups affect the binding of the molecule to the $GABA_A$ receptor and so can modulate the pharmacological properties, the potency of the effect, and the pharmacokinetic conditions (duration of the effect, distribution, etc.).

BZDs have proven to be excellent drugs for the known pharmacological properties they present, as shown in **Table 1**.

In humans, benzodiazepines are also recognized to have anterograde amnestic effects, providing amnesia for events that occur subsequent to the administration of the drug [6]. Another important use they have is in alcohol withdrawal syndrome (AWS). They are generally considered to provide no analgesia.

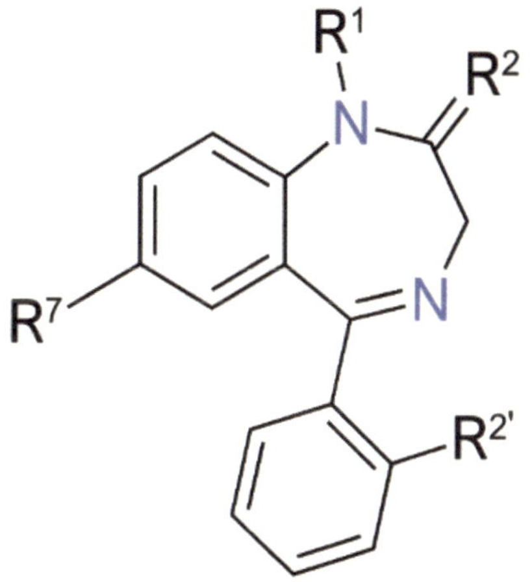

Figure 1. BZD structure.

Action	Clinical uses
Anxiolytic	Anxiety and panic/phobias, alcohol withdrawal
Hypnotic	Insomnia
Muscle relaxant	Muscle spasms, spasticity caused by CNS pathologies
Anticonvulsive	Attacks caused by drug intoxications, some forms of epilepsy
Amnesic	Intraoperatively or pre-surgery medication

Table 1. Principal actions and uses of BZDs [5].

It is important to note that the variation of the dose changes the effects: a hypnotic BZD administered in low doses produces anxiety-relieving effects, whereas a BZD marketed as an antianxiety drug at higher doses induces sleep.

1.2. Mechanism of action

To understand their mechanism of action, it is necessary to know the physiology and function of the *gamma*-aminobutyric acid (GABA) neurotransmitter. They are neurotransmitters in the central nervous system (CNS) that increment or decrease the excitability of neurons and so regulate the brain activity. GABA functions as the principal inhibitory neurotransmitter, and BZDs potentiate that function.

The GABAA receptor is a protein complex located in the synapses of neurons. It belongs to a family of receptors associated to ionic channels, formed by combinations of protein subunits with high selectivity for chloride ion (Cl^-). They conduct chloride ions across neuronal cell membranes. The receptor is formed by five subunits arranged around the central chloride: two alphas, two betas, and one gamma. There are also multiple isoforms of each subunit: six alpha subtypes ($\alpha_{1,2,3,4,5,6}$), four beta ($\beta_{1,2,3,4}$), three gamma ($\gamma_{1,2,3}$), and one delta (δ). These receptors are heterogeneous and can consist of different mixtures of different polypeptide classes (alpha, beta, gamma, etc.)

There are two GABA binding sites in the receptor and a single binding site for the BZDs which is located in the pairing (interphase) between an α subunit and a β subunit (**Figure 2**).

The binding of a BZD to its binding site cause an increment of the GABA affinity for its own binding site. They act as a **positive allosteric modulator**: the union of the BZD to the receptor does not alter the GABA union, but it increases the total conduction of chloride ions across the neuronal cell membrane. This increment of chloride ions leads to a hyperpolarization of the neuron and, as a result, a decrease of the neuronal activity [8].

The advantage of the BZDs comparing to other drugs that act in the same receptor and decrease the activity of neurons is that BZDs are the only drugs that give GABA more affinity for its receptor and act as an allosteric modulator. For the same reason, BZDs are not able to provide a higher activation than GABA itself, and this is what explains the elevated therapeutic index (toxic/therapeutic dose ratio), superior than barbiturates.

This last group, barbiturates, in low doses helps to maintain the chloride channel opened by acting in the GABA. However, in high doses they open directly the chloride cannel, which can lead to toxicity.

1.3. Specific BZD receptors

The BZD receptor has been classified into different types, based on α subunit isoforms and clinical effects related to each type [8, 9]. In addition, each BZD has different affinity to the $GABA_A$ receptor and its subunits:

- The BZ_1 receptor contains the α1 subunit isoform, which represents approximately the 60% of the $GABA_A$ receptors. This receptor is highly concentrated in the cortex, thalamus, and cerebellum, and it is responsible for sedative effects and anterograde amnesia, explaining this frequent side effect in the most of the BZDs.
- The BZ_2 receptor contains the α_2 isoform, and the BZ_3 contains the α_3 isoform. Although the BZ_2 is a widespread receptor, it is believed that those located in the spinal cord and motor neurons largely mediate myorelaxant effect, such as BZ_3 receptor, and those located in the limbic system are responsible for the anxiolytic effect.

The different effects of the BZDs are explained by their interaction and binding with the different receptors (the isoform, the affinity of the binding, and the location of the receptor in the CNS). According to this, all the effects should be expected for those BZDs that interact indiscriminately with all the receptors. Others, nonbenzodiazepines or Z-drugs, for example, only interact with one type of receptor (BZ1 in this case) so they are going to be used with more specificity.

1.4. Chemical structure and structure-activity relationship (SAR)

As introduced before, BZDs have a cyclic structure that includes one benzene cycle (*benzo*) plus a heterocycle where two atoms are nitrogen (*–diaza-*) normally in 1 and 4 positions but which

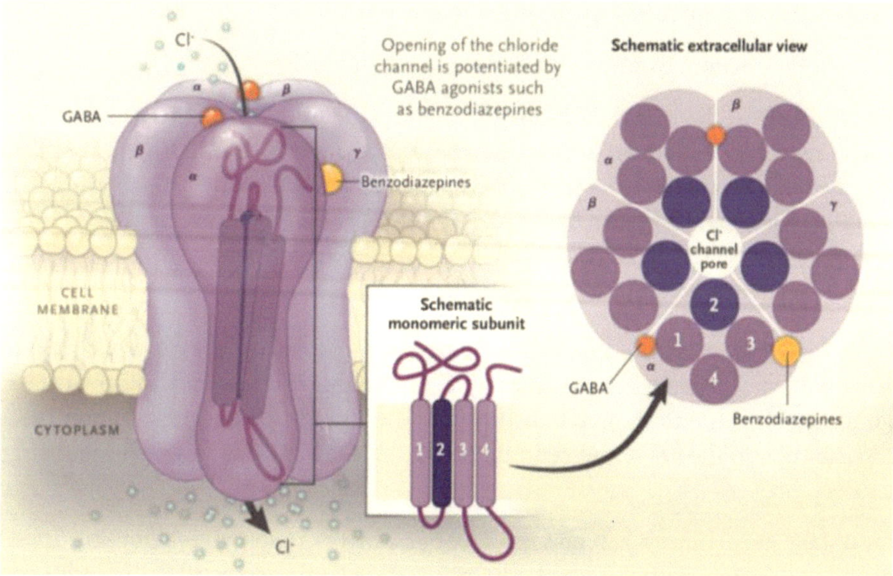

Figure 2. The $GABA_A$ receptor. On the left, a side complete view of the receptor: the subunits and the chloride ion channel, with the BZDs binding sites. On the right, a top view of the receptor, illustrating the most common combination of α, β, and γ subunits [7].

can also be in 1,5 or 2,3. Normally the benzodiazepines used in clinical are 1,4-dinitrogenated systems.

By analyzing the structure, we can see the substitutions at the different positions of and the consequences that have on the activity:

- Substitution at position 1: ↑ Activity by alkylation (prodrug). Example: *diazepam*
- Substitution at position 2: Electronegative atom

  (O or N) derived from carboxyl → first generation of BZDs. Although it can also be non-substituted. Example: medazepam

- Substitution at position 3: If it is not substituted or has an –OH: ↑ polarity → glucuronidation → faster elimination. Example: lorazepam
- Benzene ring at position 5: Optimal for activity.
  - Substituted in *ortho* by **Cl, F**: ↑ activity (electron-attracting group). Example: *flurazepam* (F) and *clonazepam* (Cl).
  - Replaced by another cycle. Example: cyclohexenyl (tetrazepam).
- Substitution at position 7: Establish the potency.

  Favorable position to ↑ activity, specially by an electron-attracting group: $CF_3 > NO_2 > Br > Cl > OCH_3 > R$.

  - NO_2: Hypnotic action.

Example: clonazepam, nitrazepam, and lormetazepam.

- X: Anxiolytic action. Example: lorazepam and alprazolam.

Any substitution on the other positions (6, 8, and 9) may decrease the activity. There are others who are fused with triazole or imidazole ring and so producing *triazolobenzodiazepines* or *imidazolobenzodiazepine* (or diazolobenzodiazepines), respectively [10]. From a chemical structure point of view, BZDs can be divided in three groups (**Figures 3** and **4**).

1.5. Pharmacokinetics and pharmacodynamics

Some of the pharmacokinetics properties change in function of the side groups (R) of each BZD. That will be decisive when prescribing them. Normally this family of drugs is taken by oral administration due to its good absorption. The intravenous administration presents a quick distribution to the brain and central nervous system, but it is reserved for emergencies like acute seizures.

BZDs and their metabolites are highly protein bound (90% union with albumin). These compounds are widely distributed in the body and preferentially accumulated in lipid-rich areas

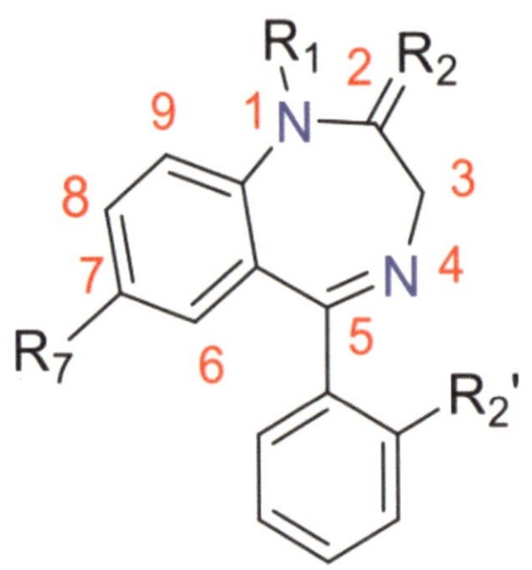

Figure 3. Compound numbering.

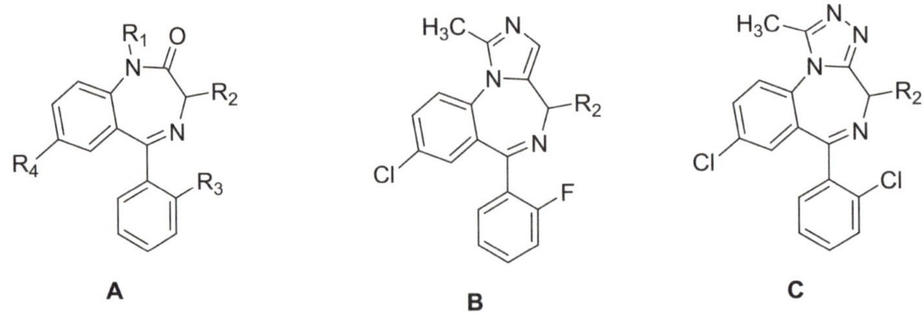

Figure 4. General structure of various BZDs: (A) 5-Aryl-1,4-benzodiazepine; (B) *midazolam*, a diazolobenzodiazepine; and (C) *triazolam*, a triazolobenzodiazepine [11].

such as the central nervous system and adipose tissue. It is important to mention that the major factor in predicting amnesia risk is lipid solubility: the greater the lipid solubility, the greater the risk of amnesia. BZDs with high lipid solubility have higher absorption rates and faster onset of clinical effects than BZDs with low lipid solubility [8]. Most BZDs are metabolized by the cytochrome P450 enzymes (phase I) by oxidation, hydroxylation, or dealkylation and after conjugated with glucuronide or sulfate (phase II). At the end, the urine excretes them almost entirely.

Some BZDs produce active metabolites during the process, as they are administered in a prodrug form. This supposes an important consideration when prescribing these agents. For example, *diazepam*, a long-acting BZD, produces the active metabolites *oxazepam*, *desmethyldiazepam*, and *temazepam*. A classification of the BZDs exists in basis of their half-live time for elimination, an estimation of the time needed to reduce the drug concentration in the plasma by half. After 5–7 h post-administration, a drug is eliminated from the body [8].

These previous reasons should be considered when administering BZDs in the elderly and in the patients with preexisting hepatic diseases: the metabolites further increase the duration of drug action, which can also have variations in the elimination half-life.

2. Classification of BZDs

BZDs are classified in terms of their elimination half-life in short-acting, intermediate-acting, or long-acting (**Figure 5**):

- Short-acting. Elimination half-life <5 h (*midazolam* and *triazolam*). Mainly used as hypnotic for their quick sleep onset. They have few residual effects and can cause rebound insomnia when disruption, as well as amnesia and dependence problems.
- Intermediate-acting. Elimination half-life 5–24 h, normally they are used for anxiety purposes. Might have next-day residual effects if used as hypnotic (alprazolam, lorazepam, lormetazepam).
- Long-acting. Elimination half-life >24 h, arriving to 100 h in diazepam. They present risk of accumulation, especially in the elderly or patients with metabolism disease (diazepam, clorazepate).

A huge number of BZDs have been synthetized over the years, but only a few had shown improved efficacy and are actually used in clinical. Today, approximately 35 benzodiazepine derivatives exist, 21 of which have been approved internationally by clinical use [7].

2.1. Abuse and dependence: problem presentation

BZDs became one of the most frequently prescribed drugs in the world around the 1970s, even though the potential abuse and dependence was quickly detected. As a result of many concerns about misuse, BZDs were placed on the Food and Drug Administration (FDA) restricted drug list in 1975. It was not until the 1980s that the dependence occurring with these drugs was confirmed, after several clinical trials and after many declarations coming from not only patients but also from clinicians. Despite recommendations of a treatment no longer than 4 weeks, many of

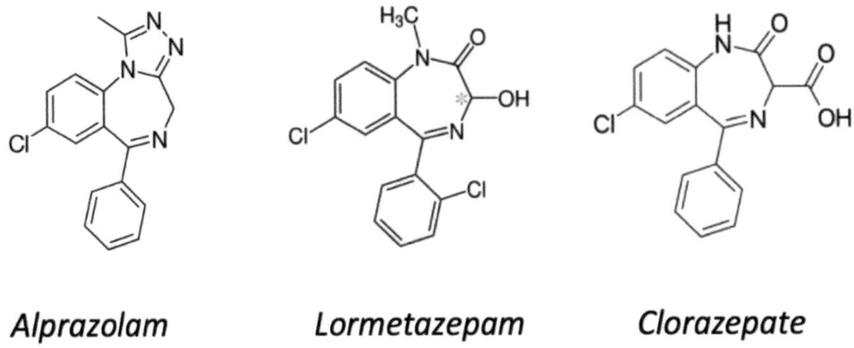

Figure 5. Examples of 1,4-benzodiazepines.

them continued to prescribe them for months or even years. Their use gradually declined after the mid-1980s as a result of growing information and concerns, and also with the discovery of other antianxiety medications like the selective serotonin reuptake inhibitors (SSRIs), which proved to be safer and more effective than BZDs. In fact, the total BZD use increased from 1999 to 2014, mainly caused by the augmentation of the long-term inappropriate users [12].

Intentional abusers of BZD usually have other substance abuse problems. Benzodiazepines are usually a secondary drug of abuse, used mainly to augment the "high" received from another drug or to offset the adverse effects of other drugs. Few cases of addiction originated from legitimate use of benzodiazepines. On August 31, 2016, FDA issued a drug safety communication about serious risks, including death, when opioid pain or cough medicines are combined with benzodiazepines. The safety announcement warned that "health care professionals should limit prescribing opioid pain medicines with benzodiazepines... only to patients for whom alternative treatment options are inadequate" [13].

The pharmacological dependence derived from a BZD, which is normally manifested in withdrawal symptoms when the treatment is suddenly interrupted, can happen even from a legitimate use. This response, caused by the constant action of drug after a long time, can be avoided, for example, with dose tapering and/or medication switching [14].

2.2. Adverse effects

In general, BZD are well-tolerated drugs if the use and administration are correct. The toxicological profile of BZDs is similar between compounds, although the frequency and gravity of the reactions can be different. In most of the cases, adverse reactions are a prolongation of the pharmacological action that affects the CNS.

- Frequent: somnolence (half of the patients experiment it during the first days of treatment), sedation, ataxia (especially in the elderly), fatigue, and anterograde amnesia (difficulty to remember recent facts)
- Occasionally: dizziness, headache, depression, confusion, and dysphasia
- Exceptionally: rush or urticaria, pruritus, and visual and/or audition alterations

They can also produce problems in psychomotor performances (driving, incoordination, sometimes causing falls). There is sufficient evidence from epidemiologic and experimental studies to establish a strong causal connection between benzodiazepine and also Z-drug use to motor vehicle accidents, falls, and fractures as a consequence of psychomotor impairment [15]. In addition, taking into account their pharmacological properties, benzodiazepines can cause muscular hypotonia and respiratory difficulties, especially in patients presenting a respiratory deficiency.

The intensity of the effects depends on the doses and is worst in patients with hepatic alterations and in the elderly. The physiological changes of aging in the liver result in prolonged clearance of drugs: by decreasing the metabolism, the half-life elimination increases. BZDs are eliminated slowly from the body, so repeated doses over a prolonged period can result in significant accumulation in fatty tissues. Thus, some symptoms of overmedication (impaired thinking, disorientation, confusion, slurred speech) can appear over time [8].

The side effects of BZDs are increased when paired with other drugs such as barbiturates, alcohol, narcotics, or tranquilizers. BZDs potentiate the sedative effects of opioids and are the most common combination in polydrug users, along with alcohol [6]. The risk of fatality via respiratory or nervous system depression from BZD overdose is barely inexistent, but if they are involved with other agents known to cause CNS and respiratory depressions, especially alcohol or opioids, the risk of harm substantially increases.

Over the past few years, biomedical literature has emerged raising a tentative link between benzodiazepine and/or Z-drug exposure with adverse outcomes such as respiratory disease exacerbation, infections, dementia, pancreatitis, and cancer. Doubt persists in the biomedical community regarding this relatively new safety accusation against these drugs by pharmacoepidemiologic researchers.

Based on the Hill criteria for causation, a list of the possible adverse outcome associations is indicated in **Table 2**.

	Traffic accidents	**Falls leading to fractures**	**Dementia**	**Infections**	**Pancreatitis**	**Respiratory worsening**	**Cancer**
Consistency	+	+	±	±	±	–	±
Strength	+	+	+	±	+	±	±
Temporality	+	+	–	+	–	–	–
Specificity	–	–	–	–	–	–	–
Dose–response	+	+	±	–	±	–	±
Coherence	+	+	±	±	–	±	–
Experimental evidence	+	+	–	±	–	±	–
Analogy	+	+	–	–	±	+	–

+ criteria fulfilled, ± criteria partially fulfilled or arguable either way, – criteria not fulfilled.

Table 2. Criteria for BZD/Z-drug adverse events [16].

There is a lack of evidence to prove causality between BZD and Z-drugs to any of these conditions due to insufficient and conflicting evidence from both epidemiologic and experimental studies, except for fall leading to fractures, which has already been proved [15]. Anyway, there are reasons to associate them: there are clinical studies that are in process to verify it or that are proposed for future research about the subject.

3. Synthesis of benzodiazepines

The first BZD, serendipitously founded, was *chlordiazepoxide,* and its synthesis started after the synthesis of the *quinazoline-N-oxide*3 as indicated in **Scheme 1**. From the 2-aminobenzophenone, the synthesis of BZDs can be raised as indicated below:

The 2-aminobenzophenone is treated with hydroxylamine to obtain the oxime **1**. The oxime can exist in the form of two stereoisomers *Z* and *E*, the stereoisomer *E* being the most stable due to steric problems. The reaction of this compound with *chloroacetylchloride* gives the chloroacetamide, which by treatment with NaOH leads to the found benzodiazepine-*N*-oxide **5**. The intramolecular cyclization reaction proceeds through the nitrogen atom of the oxime. The resulting *N*-oxide function can be reduced by treatment with PCl_3.

By treating this *quinazoline-N-oxide* with secondary amines (HNRR), a tertiary amine was obtained as an expected compound for the nucleophilic substitution **(6)**. However, by treating it with a primary amine: *methylamine* (CH_3NH_2), the result was an unexpected compound

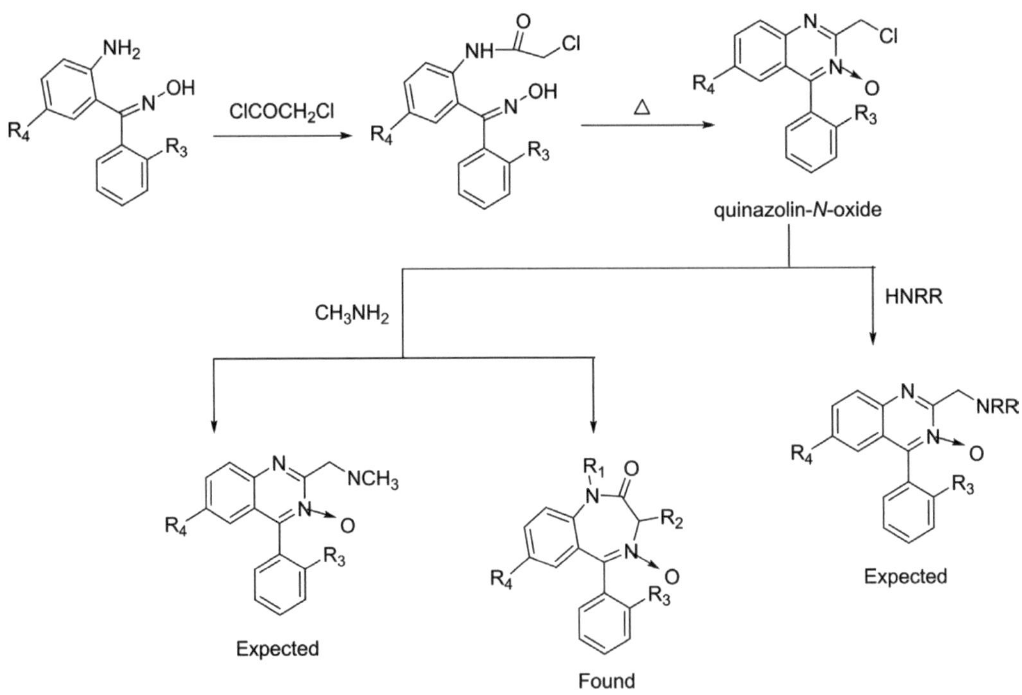

Scheme 1. Synthesis of [1, 4]-benzodiazepines [2].

http://dx.doi.org/10.5772/intechopen.79879

considered a derivative from *1,4-benzodiazepine-N[4]-oxide (9)*. An addition reaction in the carbon C-2 of the quinazoline was produced, with a rearrangement of the 6-atom ring (quinazoline) to a 7-atom ring (benzodiazepine) as a consequence (**Scheme 2**).

The reaction was generalized for other primary amines, but none of the new obtained products was better than *chlordiazepoxide* after all. Later they found that *N*-oxide group was not essential for the biological action.

Thus, new anxiolytic drugs such as *diazepam, bromazepam, or nitrazepam* were found, widely used nowadays.

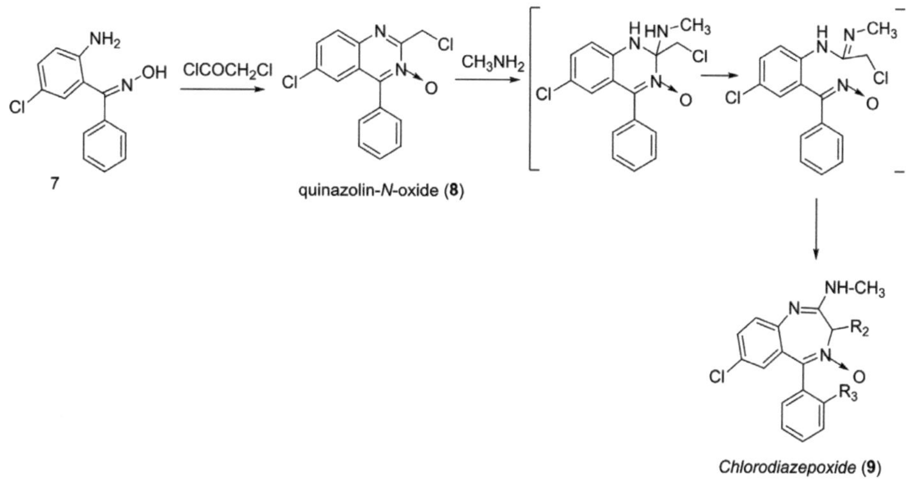

Scheme 2. Mechanism preparation of *chlordiazepoxide* [17].

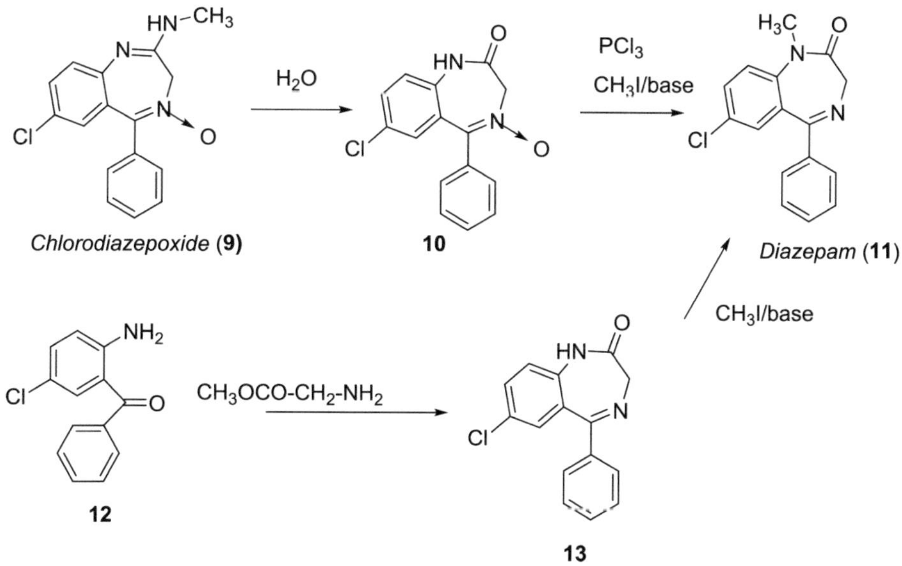

Scheme 3. Metabolism and synthesis of *diazepam* [2].

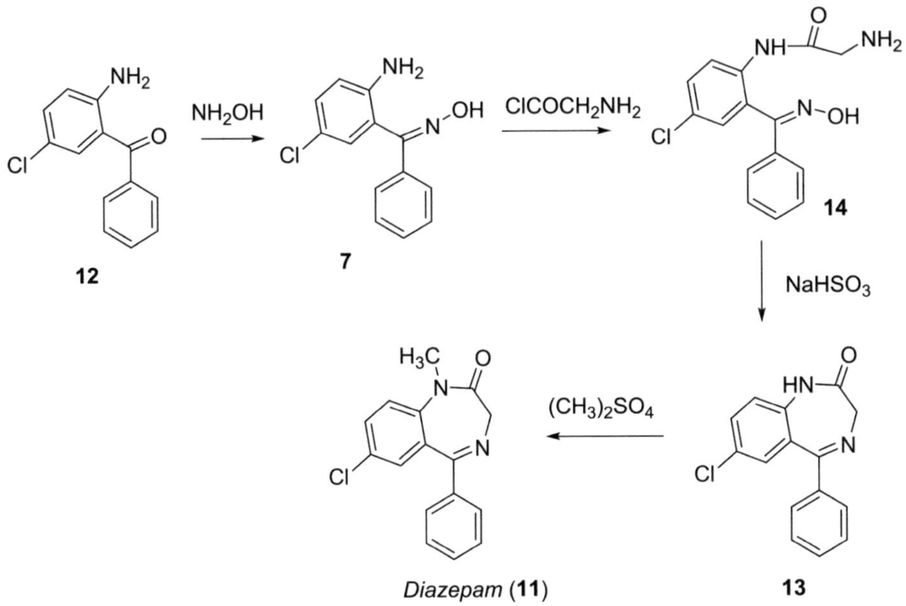

Scheme 4. Alternative synthesis of *diazepam* [17].

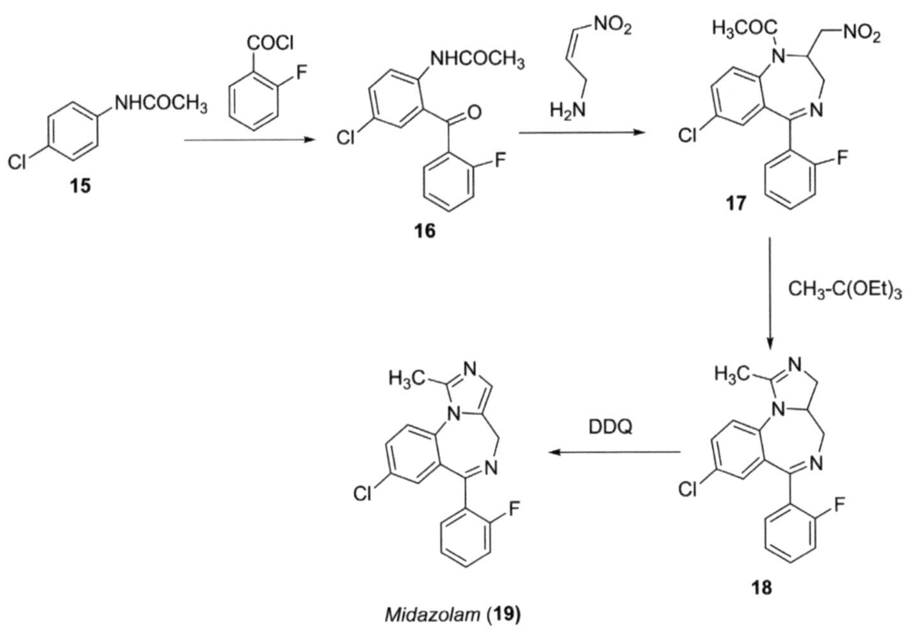

Scheme 5. Synthesis of *midazolam* [18].

In the first line of the previous scheme, we can see how *diazepam* is formed by metabolism of *chlordiazepoxide* (**9**) (**Scheme 3**). The first step is an oxidative deamination then the reduction of *N*-oxide **10** with PCl_3 following with *N*-alkylation using CH_3I/base, which introduces a methyl group by nucleophilic substitution, obtaining the metabolite *diazepam*.

Scheme 3 shows also an alternative synthesis for *diazepam* from ketone **12**, starting with a cyclization of the corresponding keto-aniline with methyl 2-aminoacetate. Then with CH_3-I/base again the introduction of a methyl group in the nitrogen of the amide leads to *diazepam*.

However, d*iazepam* has other alternative synthesis (**Scheme 4**). Starting with the 2-amino-5-chlorobenzophenone **12** and reacting with NH_2OH, we obtain the oxime **7**. Then by reacting with $ClCOCH_2NH_2$, this group is introduced by addition of the amino group to the carbonyl, ready for the next steps: a cyclization by dehydration with $NaHSO_3$ and the introduction of a methyl group to obtain the *diazepam* (**11**).

The last scheme is midazolam's synthesis, as an example of a *diazolobenzodiazepine*.

Midazolam can be prepared from 4-chloroacetanilide (**15**) by treatment with 2-fluorobenzoyl chloride. The obtained ketone **16** is treated with 3-nitro-2-propanamine to obtain the intermediate benzodiazepine **17**. Next, the nitro derivative **17** is reduced, and ethyl orthoformate is added to obtain the tricyclic system **18**. Finally, the oxidation of **18** with DDQ (2,3-dichloro-5,6-dicyanobenzoquinone) leads to *midazolam* (**Scheme 5**).

4. Traditional uses and new discoveries

When research scientists could finally give an explanation for the mechanism of action to understand the results they were obtaining with BZDs, a breakthrough happened, not only in the knowledge of anxiety but also in other central phenomena such as sleep problems or seizures.

An important advance was concerning the barbiturates. Barbiturate abuse—both prescription and illicit—peaked in the 1970s, but by the late 1980s, barbiturates had been largely replaced by benzodiazepines for treatment of anxiety and insomnia due to safety issues [19]. BZDs proved to be effective for the same purposes but with a superior therapeutic index and lower risk to cause respiration depression, the principal serious adverse effect that made barbiturates a dangerous drug with restricted uses.

Generally, it can be considered that all BZDs that are actually used in clinical are anxiolytics in low doses and hypnotic in high doses. Pharmacokinetic properties are what differentiate each compound and what define the use. Furthermore, all the treatments with BZDs should be short term due to their probability to cause tolerance and dependence problems.

4.1. Anxiolitics

Back then, the explanation of BZDs' mechanism of action supposed an important discovery in the knowledge of anxiety, which the biological basis was not completely clear.

BZDs should be seen as a symptom treatment for this condition, to facilitate the patients' adaptation or reaction to a difficult situation in their everyday life but not as a first-choice anxiety treatment. Treating anxiety should be a personalized combination of drugs and psychotherapy during the period of time the patient need, and BZDs should be only used for sporadic moments.

Nowadays there are other drugs as a first choice for anxiety treatment that does not present any long-term use problem and that show good results (SSRIs or SNRIs). Anyway, BZDs are indicated in several anxieties for short-term management of anxiety. They can be also used as an adjunct in treatment for panic disorders (PD), generalized anxiety disorders (GAD), and social anxiety disorders (SAD) as adjuncts to SSRIs for treatment of obsessive–compulsive disorder or as adjuncts to antipsychotics for treatment of acute mania or agitation [8, 20].

The BZDs used for relieving anxiety are the ones with long half-lives, which are converted in other active metabolites that also have long half-lives. According to this, we achieve continuous drug concentrations and therefore a long duration of action and effects. Some of these drugs are *alprazolam, bromazepam, oxazepam, clorazepate, diazepam,* and *lorazepam.*

It is important to note that even if the different compounds are in the same family and are used for the same objectives, they have different potencies, and the doses can notably range between compounds. For example, alprazolam is presented in 0.25, 0.5, 1, and 2 mg doses; a dose of 0.5 mg of alprazolam is equivalent to 10 mg of diazepam. That can lead to administration mistakes if there is a change between these two BZDs, for example.

4.2. Hypnotics

The quality of a hypnotic drug is not judged only on sleep but also on the state of the subject on awakening and during day, somnolence or not, on the possibility of adverse effects, etc. BZDs are used for hypnotic purposes because they increase the total sleep time by decreasing the time to fall asleep and the number of awakenings. However, the architecture of sleep is significantly altered [21]: it is composed by four non-REM stages (of which the 1 and 2 are considered light-sleep phases, while 3 and 4 phases are associated with deep sleep) and a REM stage. BZDs reduce the 3 and 4 stages and decrease the REM sleep stage, known as "the most restful phase of sleep" [22]. That could be translated, in a long-term, as a worsening of sleep quality [23].

They are useful for treating occasional insomnia, in short treatments (they must be used only for 2–4 weeks) or with an intermittent use. The most used for this objective are *lormetazepam, triazolam, nitrazepam, loprazolam, flunitrazepam,* and *estazolam.*

Either short-acting or long-acting, BZDs can be used:

- To treat insomnia characterized by a difficulty of falling sleep, this BZD will have a rapid onset and a short duration of action, with the objective to quickly achieve higher concentrations. Among hypnotic benzodiazepines, triazolam is one, which has the fastest effect, but it also causes adverse effects such as amnesia and dependence problems.
- In other cases, when the patient tends to awake in the middle of the night and is not able to continue sleeping, intermediate or long action BZD is more useful.

The duration of the action must be adapted to the sleep period: if it is too short, it might be insufficient, and if it is too long, the patient can have residual insomnia on the next day.

In many cases, there is no need of pharmacological treatment for insomnia. The following recommendations are proposed: to change the sleep habits, to avoid caffeine late in the day, or to limit the electronics devices (mobile phone, TV) in the bedroom. Exercise can often help to promote a more restful sleep as well. All these options must be tried before starting a BZD treatment.

4.3. Muscle relaxant

Benzodiazepines such as *diazepam* may be used short term as muscle relaxants reducing the tone of skeletal muscle. The myorelaxant effect is mediated through α_2-containing receptors (and α_3 in a less extent) in the spinal cord and motor neurons [8]. They can also help relieve the pain of the spasticity caused by other CNS pathologies. High doses are used: 2–10 mg even 4 times a day, depending on the severity and the patient's age, so adverse effects must be considered.

4.4. Anticonvulsive

Clonazepam is the benzodiazepine most frequently used for long-term control and prevention of chronic seizure disorders. For this purpose, it is used at high doses to achieve high brain concentrations. However, in general BZDs are not the first choice for long-term treatment for epilepsy due to the tolerance and dependence problems that they present. Traditional types of seizure treatments should be used in first line for epilepsy.

Despite that, all BZDs have anticonvulsant properties especially for seizures caused by toxic agents or due to alcohol withdrawal syndrome. For most types of acute or prolonged seizures or *status epilepticus*, an intravenous or rectal benzodiazepine would be the treatment of first choice.

4.5. Amnesics

It is important to note that in the perioperative setting, BZDs are used specifically for their amnesic properties, but in nearly all other instances, amnesia is an undesired side effect.

Their use can be advantageous as an adjunct to anesthesia to induce relaxation and amnesia (procedural memory loss) in cases of outpatient surgery or procedure that allows the patient to return home the same day, for example, endoscopy or colonoscopy, which can cause discomfort to the patients.

Intravenous *midazolam* is normally the preference in these cases due to its rapid onset and short duration of action. However, recent researchers have found that sublingual *alprazolam* is as effective and safe as oral midazolam for sedation during esophagogastroduodenoscopy (EGD): *they were similar in reducing procedural anxiety, and patients had similar tolerance and satisfaction with both treatments; however, sublingual alprazolam was accompanied with less pain/discomfort during EGD* [24].

4.6. Other uses

BZDs can be used in patients in the intensive care unit (ICU) in those with mechanical ventilation or those with acute pain, although they should be used carefully because of the possible respiratory depression in some cases.

- They are proved to be first-line choice in AWS treatment. AWS results in people who are dependent on alcohol and either stopped drinking or reduced their alcohol consumption. Severe forms of AWS may be associated with generalized seizures, hallucinations, and delirium tremens, which can be fatal [25]. BZDs have proved to be the best studied and most effective drugs, especially to prevent severe symptoms and particularly the risk of seizures and delirium tremens. The most used oral BZDs for this pathology are diazepam, chlordiazepoxide, and lorazepam.

- BZDs can be used for abreaction, a technique applied to recover memories.

5. A new discovery: BET inhibitors

A few years ago, BZDs started to be investigated by their possible action as BET protein inhibitors. These families of proteins (bromo- and extra-terminal domain, BET) are epigenetic reader proteins, involved in transcription regulation and chromatin remodeling. Each protein contains two domains (D1 and D2) that bind acetylated lysine on histones H3 and H4. This bind is produced in the hydrophobic pocket of BET by hydrogen bonding, where researchers found high-affinity small molecule ligands that block the binding with the histones. These BET protein inhibitors are the first successful example of inhibition of epigenetic readers, and they offer the opportunity to target cancer drivers, for example, the family of proto-oncogenes *MYC*. Thus, BET inhibitor treatment of cancer cells dependent on the oncogene c-*MYC* can result in significant antiproliferative and cytotoxic effects [25].

In view of the results, at least 10 BET inhibitors are in clinical trials today for the treatment of a range of hematological cancers (including leukemia, lymphoma, and myeloma), certain solid tumors, and atherosclerosis [26]. Most of these molecules are structurally based on the BZD family and have their pharmacological properties.

On November 2017, a new study was published concerning the *design, synthesis, and biological activity of 1,2,3-triazolobenzodiazepines BET inhibitors* [27]. Starting from the previous recent discoveries, they focused in testing if the different molecules had acetyl lysine mimicking activity. Based on the bromodomain-binding framework, they developed a 1,2,3-*triazolobenzodiazepine* with the optimal conditions for hydrogen bounding: a diazepine ring for protection and high affinity with asparagine.

The synthesis of **25** (**Scheme 6**) was carried out in the following way: first formation of the diarylamine **21** from the 1,2-diiodobenzene **20** and the aniline by means of a Buchwald cross-coupling reaction. Then, an introduction of an alkyne under Sonogashira coupling reaction conditions. The acylation of **22** with the 2-chloroacetyl chloride leads to **23**. Subsequently the addition of sodium azide to **23** allows a 1,3-dipolar cycloaddition cascade that leads directly to the *triazolobenzodiazepine* **24** by heating at 150°C. The yield of this step was low (13%). Finally, the reduction of carbonyl group with BH_3 provided **25**.

They assessed this compound by a binding assay (*AlphaScreen*), and it showed good activity against all bromodomains. After that, they optimize it and expand the series, obtaining a range of analogs.

BET inhibitors have been shown to have a remarkable effect on certain primary cells and cell lines, consequently of downregulation of oncogenes like c-*MYC*. From all of the analogs, and after the tests were done, they selected two of these compounds, both with excellent selectivity in BET domains, and tested them against a cancer cell panel to study their antileukemic effects.

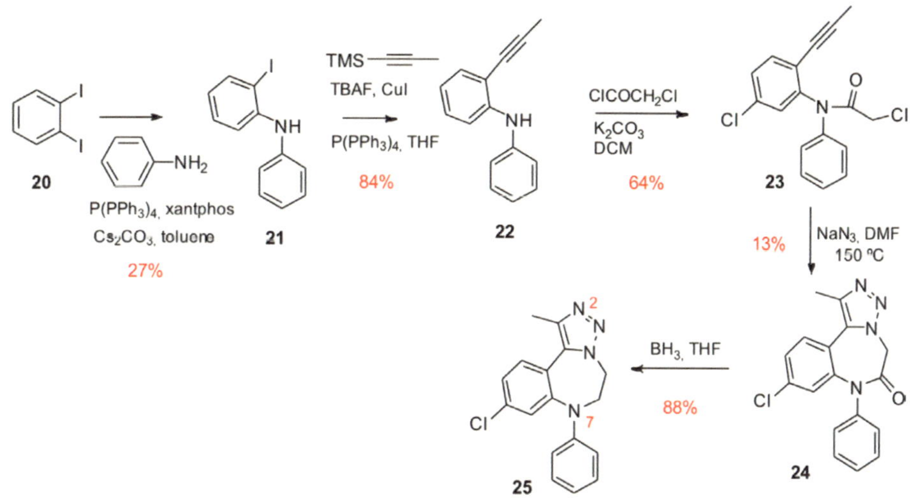

Scheme 6. Synthesis of 7 (1,2,3-*triazolobenzodiazepine*) [27].

They showed potent antiproliferative activity in some specific leukemia and downregulation of oncogene *MYC*. They also tested them on primary mouse osteosarcoma (OS) cells: both compounds inhibited proliferation of primary OS cell types, showing the utility of 1,2,3-*triazolobenzodiazepine* derivatives in cancer studies.

This new line of study shows a different and interesting use for BZDs that needs to continue to be developed according to the actual interest in the different lines of cancer treatment research. It is an example of how drugs that already exists for a determinate purpose can become the main source for a study with very different new indications.

5.1. Analysis of the reasons that lead to abuse and addiction

Nowadays, BZDs are mostly used for symptomatic treatment of anxiety and/or insomnia, anesthesia, and AWS. Many BZDs received FDA approval for the treatment of "anxiety states" or "anxiety disorders." Therefore, BZD treatment represents an off-label use (without FDA disease-specific approval) for most mental disorders.

Serotonergic agents (SSRIs or serotonin and norepinephrine reuptake inhibitors [SNRIs]) are the first-line pharmacologic treatments for anxiety disorders. These antidepressants typically take 4–6 weeks before they exert clinical effect, even more in the treatment of anxiety symptoms. When this treatment is initiated, it is typical to co-administer BZDs [28].

Moreover, antidepressants are not necessarily effective at starting doses. During titration to an effective dose (by increasing it in a gradual way), a patient can remain symptomatic. Consequently, it can be months before anxiety relieves because of the antidepressant treatment. Theoretically, BZDs are commonly used as adjuncts during the first few weeks of starting a serotonergic agent with the hopes that once a therapeutic dose is achieved, the BZD can be discontinued.

Unfortunately, there is no evidence to support this practice. This was verified in a cohort's study performed between 2001 and 2004 to patients with recent depression diagnosis and with no previous treatment. No significant differences were found between the group that only was taking antidepressant and the group that simultaneously started both antidepressant and BZD [29].

Despite conventional knowledge, BZDs do not make SSRIs more effective when prescribed simultaneously. There are no long-term benefits, but there is a long-term risk of physical dependence (tolerance and/or withdrawal) when these drugs are associated at the beginning of the treatment. Moreover, it is frequently for patients to continue BZDs long term in the presence or absence of the antidepressant. Despite many clinicians intending to interrupt them after the 4–6 weeks (when SSRIs begin to have their therapeutic effect), 12% of patients receiving this treatment and trialed at the study previously mentioned to continue BZDs for over 6 months—sometimes in the absence of SSRIs—likely indicating the difficulty of discontinuing BZDs once started [29, 20].

Despite these mentioned factors, the rate of physicians prescribing this way has not stopped growing in the last 25 years [28]. Because of the risks associated with BZD, this practice (simultaneous new use at antidepressant initiation) requires careful consideration.

The only mental disorders—not including alcohol/sedative-hypnotic withdrawal—for which there is an evidence basis for BZD treatment are PD, GAD, social anxiety disorder (SAD), and insomnia. For these four conditions, BZDs have only demonstrated efficacy for short-term durations (less than 2–4 weeks) and for treatment-resistant cases. Even for those conditions, which there are proofs of efficacy, there is no evidence for benefit in long-term treatment [20].

Nevertheless, BZDs are frequently overprescribed for other indications for which there is no evidence of efficacy, to individuals who have contraindicated comorbid conditions, for longer periods than are recommended, and before other first- and second-line treatments are tried or offered.

Apart from these four previously mentioned, there are no other mental disorders with an evidence basis for BZD treatment. To the contrary, this treatment in post-traumatic stress disorders (PTSD) is particularly concerning because BZDs have not proved to possess preventative value and may actually increase the risk in 2–5 times of developing PTSD among the patients with trauma. Moreover, PTSD is commonly comorbid with conditions that are contraindicated for BZDs (substance use disorders, traumatic brain injury, depression, etc.), and BZDs can inhibit trauma-focused psychotherapy by inhibiting the cognitive processing, which is extremely necessary for a good recovery [30].

It is common in many disorders to find patients receiving treatment not supported by evidence-based clinical practice guidelines (CPGs). Though the only FDA-approved medications for PTSD are *sertraline* and *paroxetine* (both antidepressants), of PTSD patients receiving pharmacotherapy: 65–90% receive antidepressants, 37–74% receive sedative-hypnotics (including BZDs), and 21–34% receive antipsychotics [20]. In fact, most of CPGs strongly recommend against the use of BZDs for PTSD, such as the guideline done by the Department of Veterans Affairs/Department of Defense (VA/DOD) [31].

Psychotherapy is the gold standard treatment for anxiety, while medications are generally considered adjunctive: only serotonergic agents (SSRI and SNRI) are considered first-line pharmacologic monotherapies [32]. The evaluation of the recovery should be based on the improvement of the normal functioning and not only based on the results of the sedation, which often does not relate with the patients' improvement. A variety of evidence-based treatments might be considered previous to initiating BZD treatment if there is not a strong evidence of efficacy. In many cases of anxiety, psychotherapy or support would be advised, instead of starting a treatment with a high potential of risk.

An other reason that should be considered when talking about possible addiction is, as previously mentioned, the elevated percentage of patients who continue to use BZDs for long term or self-medication. Even when the prescription instructions are followed, these drugs normally present difficulties when discontinued, mostly due to their properties such as the quick onset and relief of the symptoms that are likely to cause addiction.

To help prevent abuse and diversion of BZDs, prescribers should use appropriate precautions, similar to those used when prescribing other controlled substances such as opioids.

5.2. "Z-drugs" or nonbenzodiazepines

As introduced before, a new type of related drugs appeared in the 1990s specifically for insomnia treatment: nonbenzodiazepines receptor agonists (NBRAs) or Z-drugs.

There are three approved: *zolpidem*, *zopiclone*, (*eszopiclone* as the active enantiomer), and *zaleplon*. They present the same mechanism of action than BZDs (facilitating the inhibitory effect of GABA) but showing more selectivity for BZ1, which affects specifically to sedation and also cause fewer adverse effects [19]. However, they do not have BZD chemical structure, not even the same between them.

The synthesis of zolpidem is proposed in **Scheme 7**. The aminomethylation of the imidazopyridine yields the 3-dimethylamino derivative **27**, which is alkylated with CH_3I to obtain the quaternary ammonium salt **28**, which is then reacted with sodium cyanide to give the corresponding nitrile **29**. The acid hydrolysis of the nitrile yields the carboxylic acid **30**, which is activated with carbonyldiimidazole (CDI) and then treated with dimethylamine excess to obtain the corresponding dimethylamide **31** (*zolpidem*) (**Figures 6** and **7**).

The adverse effects of traditional BZDs (like alteration of the sleep architecture, reduction of deep sleep (REM), and residual effects on daytime lead to dependence, tolerance, and withdrawal) have driven the development of these alternative sedative-hypnotic drugs.

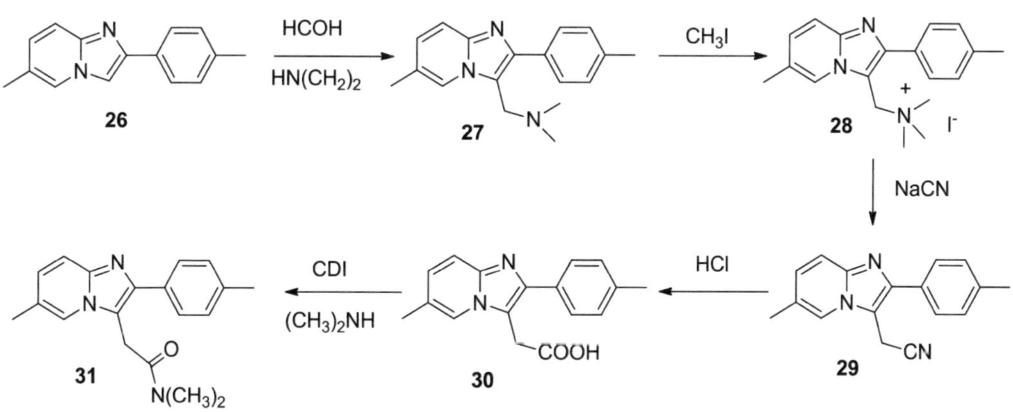

Scheme 7. Chemical structure of the three commercialized Z-drugs.

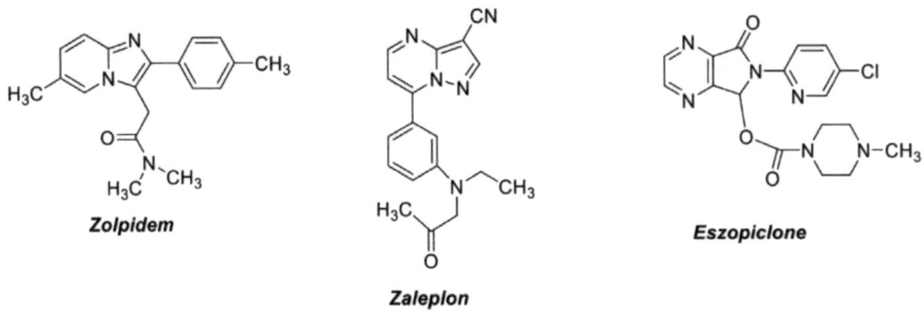

Figure 6. Synthesis of zolpidem via Mannich aminomethylation [33].

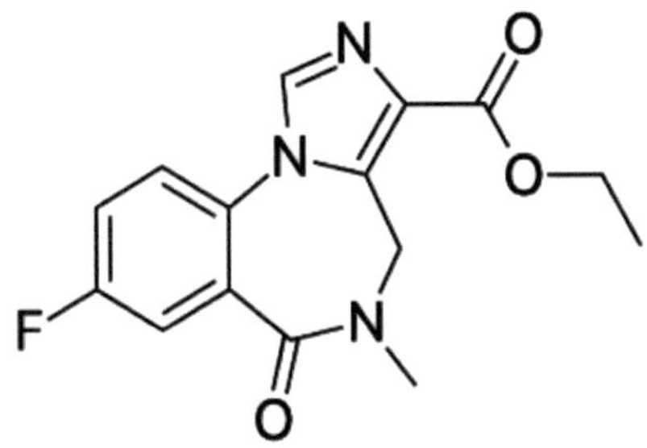

Figure 7. Flumazenil.

Z-drugs have significant hypnotic effects by reducing sleep latency and improving sleep quality, though duration of sleep may not be significantly increased. Their pharmacokinetics properties approach those of the "ideal hypnotic" with rapid onset within 30 min and short half-life (**Table 3**).

Initially clinical trials were promising due to their low adverse effects and improvements, reducing the potential of abuse. They possess short duration of action and half-life, do not disturb sleep architecture, and cause less residual effects during daytime hours, making them more clinically attractive than BZDs [22, 35].

Despite that, there are other kinds of side effects that are common among these drugs. During the first trails, the most reported side effects were nausea, dizziness, malaise, hallucination, nightmares, or agitation. Although *zolpidem* appeared to be well tolerated, there were cases of abuse, withdrawal, or tolerance in cases where the recommended dose of *zolpidem* was exceeded or with patients who had a history of substance abuse and/or a psychiatric disorder.

Later, cases of Z-drug reports causing visual hallucinations and amnesia in people with no history of mental disease appeared. Although the mechanism of action to describe these phenomena is not clear, it is speculated that *GABA receptor (α1 subunit) may be overexpressed, or they may be rapid activation after quick absorption in sensitive individuals* [36]. As seen in the reports, this is especially true for those patients with mental disease such bipolar disorder, borderline

Drug	Onset (min)	Half-life (h)	Duration of action	Insomnia indication
Zolpidem	30	1.4–4.5	Short	Sleep onset
Zolpidem ER	30	1.6–5.5	Intermediate	Sleep onset and sleep maintenance
Zaleplon	20	0.5–1	Ultrashort	Sleep onset
Eszopiclone	30	6–7	Intermediate	Sleep maintenance

ER = extended release. Due to its duration of action, *zaleplon* does not present next-day drowsiness; it can be taken within 4–5 hours of wake time without the risk of hangover effect [34].

Table 3. Principal Z-drugs and properties.

personality disorders, or drug abuse potential, because the sensitization of GABA receptors in some of these patients may predispose to the development of hallucinations [37].

Other symptoms seen in the reports are bizarre and complex behavioral effects like sleep-related complex behaviors [38], proved to be related with Z-drugs, particularly *zolpidem* [39]. There have also been some reports and posterior studies of suicidal attempts by zolpidem. In 2016 a study demonstrated a significant association between using *zolpidem* and suicide or suicide attempt in people with or without comorbid psychiatric illnesses [40].

Reports of incidents related with these drugs had increased over the years, indicating that *zolpidem* and others may not be considered as risk-free and should be carefully prescribed, dispensed, and used [19].

Studies have seen that Z-drugs usually present the same problems that of BZD: they are prescribed for longer use with excessive doses, particularly in the elderly. This fact shows a relation with the high incidence of falls and risk of hip fracture among these patients [15]. There are also studies that support the lack of demonstrable improved efficacy of Z-drugs, which causes similar rates of adverse events compared to benzodiazepines [41].

The last aspect to consider these drugs is their potential recreational use. As what happens with BZD, by mixing high doses of drug with opioids or alcohol, a major CNS depression is obtained, producing euphoric "high" symptoms with anterograde amnesia on the next day. A study carried out in 2011 showed that when *zolpidem* was ingested with other medications or ethanol, admissions to the ICU were highly common. Despite its reported safety, these overdoses often required ICU admissions, which were results of the association with other drugs and/or alcohol [42].

5.3. Tolerance, dependence, and withdrawal syndrome

Despite BZDs' successful use, tolerance was rapidly discovered and studied. A clinical trial in 1985 performed by the Medical College of Ohio showed the regional differences in down-regulation of brain BZD receptors using a quantitative autoradiographic method because of the chronic presence of this drug to its receptor locus [43].

Clinical experience showed that benzodiazepines are frequently used for long-term treatment, and there are many reasons for this: prescribing tradition, patient preference, difficulties associated with benzodiazepine withdrawal (even in patients taking low doses) because they have a rapid clinical onset of action, and good efficacy with few initial adverse effects. Long-term intake of a drug can induce tolerance of the secondary effects (because increased amounts are needed to achieve intoxication, or the effects are minimized with continued use) and physical dependence, a risk associated even at therapeutic doses [44]. There is no standard definition of long-term use, but the most common is 6–12 months. Tolerance to the sedating effects of benzodiazepines is rapid, but tolerance to the anxiolytic effects develops slowly and to a limited extent.

Symptoms of withdrawal after long-term benzodiazepine use usually develop faster with shorter-acting drugs (within 2–3 days) than with longer-acting drugs (within 5–10 days). This is presented by physical symptoms (spasms, weakness, muscle tension, etc.) and psychological symptoms (anxiety and panic disorders, agitation, mood changes). Seizures are also quite common, especially if the agent is discontinued abruptly. Severe withdrawal symptoms include paranoid thoughts, hallucinations, and delirium [7].

5.3.1. Intoxication and antidote

Generally, BZDs are a safe family of drugs because they present a large therapeutic index. Patients may misuse them by self-medication or by increasing the therapeutic dose for recreational purposes [45]. Real risk comes when patients combine these drugs with other substances: the combined use of alcohol and benzodiazepines increases the risk of a fatal overdose. A similar fatal interaction can occur with opioids: BZDs are often misused by high-risk opioid users and are associated with morbidity and mortality among this group.

Misuse or abuse may lead to intoxication or a withdrawal syndrome, which may be fatal. Differential diagnosis of intoxication by these drugs could be polydrug use (toxicity is highly augmented by combination with other drugs), epilepsy, agitation, alcohol withdrawal delirium or respiratory depression, among others [7].

Fortunately, overdose with benzodiazepines and Z-drugs responds to an antagonist, *flumazenil*, although it has its limitations and potential adverse effects.

This benzodiazepine antagonist, *flumazenil*, is available for the treatment of acute benzodiazepine intoxication and has been shown to reverse also the sedative effects of all three Z-drugs [35]. Actually, it is a BZD with high affinity, which is able to displace other BZDs and has very short half-life, of approximately 1 hour.

It is used for:

- BZDs or Z-drugs intoxications
- To reverse the effects of anesthesia caused by a BZD
- Diagnosis of states of coma, which have an unknown origin

However, it may not completely reverse respiratory depression, and it can provoke withdrawal seizures in patients with benzodiazepine dependence [9].

5.3.2. *Possible treatment of dependence to avoid withdrawal symptoms*

Based on several guidelines to avoid withdrawal symptoms, different steps are recommended when patients want to quit a BZD treatment. For the following recommendations, a specific guideline is consulted: *Benzodiazepines: how they work and how to withdraw* or commonly known as *The Ashton Manual* [46]. It is written by Professor C Heather Ashton, a psychopharmacologist from Newcastle, who has dedicated the majority of her career to psychotropic drugs, and especially to BZDs.

Successful withdrawal strategies should combine gradual dosage reduction and sufficient psychological support. The precise rate of withdrawal is an individual matter and should be personalized, depending on many factors including the dose and type of BZD used, the duration of use, and the personality and the will of the patient. For patients without any motivation for withdrawal and those with a severe depressive episode or other major mental disorders, stabilization might be preferable before initiating withdrawal treatment [7].

Various authors suggest optimal times from 6 to 8 weeks to several months for the duration of withdrawal, but some patients may take a year or more if they have taken BZDs in prolonged use. The best results are achieved if the patient himself is in control of the rate of withdrawal and proceeds at whatever rate he finds tolerable.

5.3.2.1. *Dose tapering*

Sedative withdrawal symptoms can be avoided by slowly tapering down the dose of the BZD over several weeks and by managing the anxiety if needed. Under any circumstances it is recommended to suddenly stop the treatment. Abrupt withdrawal, especially from high doses, can precipitate convulsions, acute psychotic or confusional states, and panic reactions [47]. The ideal situation is one where the patient, with the help of the doctor, decides together the schedule, accepting that there will be readjustments to the time according to his progress. The length of time between each dose reduction should be based on the presence and severity of withdrawal symptoms. The longer the interval between reductions, the more comfortable and safer the withdrawal would be [48].

5.3.2.2. *Switching to a long-acting BZD*

With short-acting BZDs, it is impossible to achieve a smooth decline in blood and tissue concentrations because of the way they are eliminated quickly from the body. In these cases, it is preferred to switch to a long-acting and slowly metabolized BZD such as *diazepam*. Due to its metabolites and long half-life, it is easy to decrease the concentrations in a smooth and gradual way.

The dose has a very important role: not only it has to be changed by the equivalent in *diazepam* but it also has to contemplate the properties of each BZD (if changed to an anxiolytic for a hypnotic, different symptoms can be expected). *Diazepam* is also good to switch to, because its presentation (2 or 10 mg) makes the dose adaptation easier for every patient.

As indicated before, there is an equivalence of doses between different compounds depending on the active metabolites and the potency (**Table 4**).

Benzodiazepine	Half-life (h) (active metabolite)	Oral dosages (mg)
Alprazolam (Xanax)	6–12	0.5
Clonazepam (Klonopin)	18–50	0.5
Lorazepam (Ativan)	10–20	1
Diazepam (Valium)	20–100	10
Chlordiazepoxide (Librium)	5–30	25
Clorazepate (Tranxene)	36–200	15
Oxazepam (Serax)	4–15	20

Table 4. Half-life and equivalent potencies of BZD anxiolytics [5].

Most potent drugs like *alprazolam, clonazepam,* or *lorazepam,* which has 10–20 times more potency that *diazepam,* are highly addictive; dependence develops rapidly, and they are particularly hard to leave. In addition, their dose presentations do not allow a gradual dosage reduction when withdrawal.

6. Conclusions

Concerning the prescriptions, **guidelines have failed** to reduce the prescriptions: clinicians do not always adhere to recommendations to use BZDs as hypnotics and anxiolytics only for short term and only after trying psychological therapies. It has been difficult to accept the high risk and low benefits of the long term in most of the cases.

The **equivalence of doses** between different compounds had presented difficulties, leading to incorrect and excessive dose prescriptions in many situations. Prescriptions of most potent BZDs (as *alprazolam, clonazepam, or lorazepam*) with excessive dosage are the more problematic, partly of their addictive potential and partly of their dose presentation, that does not allow a gradual dosage reduction when withdrawal.

New lines of study related with BZDs as **BET inhibitor** compounds are an interesting way to change the direction of the therapeutic uses, especially long term. Other new uses, as perioperative, are a valuable way to use an adverse effect derived from the biological activity and apply it with a clinical purpose.

After analyzing the advantages and disadvantages of the **Z-drugs**, it can be concluded that even if they are not exactly as BZD, they must be treated with the same precaution due to the amount of adverse effect reports that had appeared over the recent years.

Despite the amount of biomedical literature on BZDs and Z-drugs, there is still a need to answer vital questions relevant to their effectiveness and safety in society, for example, the possibility of irreversible effects due to extended treatment, especially those associated to new safety accusations [16].

The constant investigation concerning BZDs is an indication that the problems related with these drugs are an actual concern, not only as a medical issue but also as a social concern. On July 11, there is a "World Benzodiazepine Awareness day (W-BAD)," with the objective to educate the population, to offer support to the patients suffering from dependence, and to try to gain global awareness about the dependency this kind of drugs cause if they are not prescribed correctly, among others [49].

Author details

Elisabet Batlle, Enric Lizano, Miquel Viñas and Maria Dolors Pujol*

*Address all correspondence to: mdpujol@ub.edu

Laboratory of Pharmaceutical Chemistry, Faculty of Pharmacy, University of Barcelona, Barcelona, Spain

References

[1] Strenbachh L. The benzodiazepine story. Journal of Medicinal Chemistry. 1979;**22**:1-7

[2] Rubira E, Medicamentos R. Un Viaje a Lo Largo de la Evolución Del Descubrimiento de Farmacos. Univ Santiago de Compostela; 2008. ISBN: mkt0003358332

[3] Wick J. The history of benzodiazepines. The Consultant Pharmacist. 2013;**28**:538-548

[4] López-Muñoz F, Álamo C, García P. The discovery of chlordiazepoxide and the clinical introduction of benzodiazepines: Half a century of anxiolytic drugs. Journal of Anxiety Disorders. 2011;**25**:554-562

[5] Ashton H. History of Benzodiazepines, Psychiatric Medication Awareness Group. Available from: https://www.psychmedaware.org/HistoryBenzodiazepines.html [Accessed: February 20, 2018]

[6] Harvey R, Silverstein D, Hopper K. Small Animal Critical Care Medicine. Saint Louis: Elsevier; 2009. ISBN: 9781416025917

[7] Soyka M. Treatment of benzodiazepine dependence. The New England Journal of Medicine. 2017;**376**:1147-1157

[8] Griffin CE, Kaye AM, Bueno FR, Kaye AD. Benzodiazepine pharmacology and central nervous system–mediated effects. The Ochsner Journal. 2013;**13**:214-223

[9] Nutt DJ, Stahl SM. Searching for perfect sleep: The continuing evolution of GABAA receptor modulators as hypnotics. Journal of Psychopharmacology. 2010;**24**:1601-1612

[10] Structural activity relationships of benzodiazepines. Available from: https://egpat.com/blog/structural-activity-relationships-of-benzodiazepines [Accessed: February 23, 2018]

[11] Hagan RL. Clarification of benzodiazepine structural classes. Journal of Analytical Toxicology. 1995;**19**:58-59

[12] Kaufmann CN, Spira AP, Depp CA, Mojtabai R. Long-term use of benzodiazepines and nonbenzodiazepine hypnotics, 1999-2014. Psychiatric Services. 2018;**69**:235-238

[13] FDA Drug Safety Communication. FDA Warns About Serious Risks And Death When Combining Opioid Pain Or Cough Medicines with Benzodiazepines; Requires Its Strongest Warning. Available from: https://www.fda.gov/Drugs/DrugSafety/ucm518473.htm [accessed Feb 24, 2018]

[14] O'brien CP. Benzodiazepine use, abuse, and dependence. Journal of Clinical Psychiatry. 2005;**66**:28-33

[15] Donnelly K, Bracchi R, Hewitt J, Routledge PA, Carter B. Benzodiazepines, Z-drugs and the risk of hip fracture: A systematic review and meta-analysis. PLoS One. 2017;**12**:1-14

[16] Brandt J, Leong C. Benzodiazepines and Z-drugs: An updated review of major adverse outcomes reported on in epidemiologic research. Drugs in R&D. 2017;**17**:493-507

[17] Kleemann A, Engel J, Kutscher B, Reichert D. Pharmaceutical Substances,Syntheses, Patents and Applications of the Most Relevant APIs. 5th ed. Stuttgart/New York: G. Thieme Verlag; 2014

[18] Pozo C, Macias A, Alonso E. Reactions of 1,4-benzodiazepinic N-nitrosoamidines with tosylmethyl isocyanide: A novel synthesis of midazolam. Synthesis. 2004;**16**:2697-2703

[19] Weaver MF. Prescription sedative misuse and abuse. The Yale Journal of Biology and Medicine. 2015;**88**:247-256

[20] Guina J, Merrill B. Benzodiazepines I: Upping the care on downers: The evidence of risks, benefits and alternatives. Journal of Clinical Medicine. 2018;**7**:1-22

[21] Manconi M, Ferri R, Miano S, Maestri M, Bottasini V, Zucconi M, et al. Sleep architecture in insomniacs with severe benzodiazepine abuse. Clinical Neurophysiology. 2017;**128**:875-881

[22] Roehrs T, Roth T. Drug-related sleep stage changes: Functional significance and clinical relevance. Sleep Medicine Clinics. 2010;**5**:559-570

[23] Benzodiazepines: An effective treatment for insomnia? Available from: http://flipper.diff.org/app/items/info/5332 [Accessed: February 26, 2018]

[24] Sebghatollahi V, Tabesh E, Gholamrezaei A, Zandi A, Minakari M, Shavakhi A. Premedication with benzodiazepines for upper gastrointestinal endoscopy: Comparison between oral midazolam and sublingual alprazolam. Journal of Research in Medical Sciences. 2017;**22**:1-14

[25] Sachdeva A, Choudhary M, Chandra M. Alcohol withdrawal syndrome: Benzodiazepines and beyond. Journal of Clinical and Diagnostic Research. 2015;**9**:VE01-VE07

[26] Chaidos A, Caputo V, Karadimitris A. Inhibition of bromodomain and extra-terminal proteins (BET) as a potential therapeutic approach in haematological malignancies. Therapeutic Advances in Hematology. 2015;**6**:128-141

[27] Sharp PP, Garnier J-M, Hatfaludi T, Xu Z, Segal D, Jarman KE, et al. Design, synthesis, and biological activity of 1,2,3-triazolobenzodiazepine BET bromodomain inhibitors. ACS Medicinal Chemistry Letters. 2017;**8**:1298-1303

[28] Sánchez V, Pilar M, Macías Saint-Gerons D, de la Fuente Honrubia C, González Bermejo D, Montero Corominas D, et al. Evolución Del Uso de Medicamentos Ansiolíticos e Hipnóticos En España Durante El Período 2000-2011. Revista Española de Salud Pública. 2013;**87**:247-255

[29] Bushnell GA, Stürmer T, Gaynes BN, Pate V, Miller M. Simultaneous antidepressant and benzodiazepine new use and subsequent long-term benzodiazepine use in adults with depression. JAMA Psychiatry. 2017;**74**:747-755

[30] Bleakley S, Davies SJ. The pharmacological management of anxiety disorders. Progress in Neurology and Psychiatry. 2014;**18**:27-32

[31] VA/DoD. Veterans Affairs/Department of Defense Clinical Practice Guidelines. Management of Posttraumatic Stress Disorder and Acute Stress Reaction 2017. Available from: https://www.healthquality.va.gov/guidelines/MH/ptsd [Accessed: February 27, 2018]

[32] Clinical Practice Review for GAD | Anxiety and Depression Association of America, ADAA. Available from: https://adaa.org/resources-professionals/practice-guidelines-gad [Accessed: February 26, 2018]

[33] Castaldi G. A Process for the Preparation of 2-Phenyl-Imidazo[1,2-*a*]pyridine-3-Acetamides. EP1172364B1; 2001

[34] McQueeney M; Bostwick RJ; Howell HR. Prescription Sleep Aids for the Treatment of Insomnia. Available from: https://www.uspharmacist.com/article/prescription-sleep-aids-for-the-treatment-of-insomnia [Accessed: February 21, 2018]

[35] Gunja N. The clinical and forensic toxicology of Z-drugs. Journal of Medical Toxicology. 2013;**9**:155-162

[36] Ram D, Eiman N, Gowdappa B. Multimodal hallucination (audio visual, kinaesthetic and scenic) associated with the use of zolpidem. Clinical Psychopharmacology and Neuroscience. 2015;**13**:215-217

[37] Manfredi G, Kotzalidis GD, Lazanio S, Savoja V, Talamo A, Koukopoulos AE, et al. Command hallucinations with self-stabbing associated with zolpidem overdose. The Journal of Clinical Psychiatry. 2010;**71**:92-93

[38] Park Y-M, Shin H-W. Zolpidem induced sleep-related eating and complex behaviors in a patient with obstructive sleep apnea and restless legs syndrome. Clinical Psychopharmacology and Neuroscience. 2016;**14**:299-301

[39] Dolder CR, Nelson MH. Hypnosedative-induced complex behaviours: Incidence, mechanisms and management. CNS Drugs. 2008;**22**:1021-1036

[40] Sun Y, Lin C-C, Lu C-J, Hsu C-Y, Kao C-H. Association between zolpidem and suicide: A nationwide population-based case-control study. Mayo Clinic Proceedings. 2016; **91**:308-315

[41] Siriwardena AN, Qureshi MZ, Dyas JV, Middleton H, Orner R. Magic bullets for insomnia? Patients' use and experiences of newer (Z drugs) versus older (benzodiazepine) hypnotics for sleep problems in primary care. The British Journal of General Practice. 2008;**58**:417-422

[42] Zosel A, Osterberg EC, Mycyk MB. Zolpidem misuse with other medications or alcohol frequently results in intensive care unit admission. American Journal of Therapeutics. 2011;**18**:305-308

[43] Tietz E, Rosenbger H. Autoradiographic localization of benzodiazepine receptor downregulation. The Journal of Pharmacology and Experimental Therapeutics. 1986; **236**:284-292

[44] Busto U, Sellers EM. Pharmacologic aspects of benzodiazepine tolerance and dependence. Journal of Substance Abuse Treatment. 1991;**8**:29-33

[45] Liebrenz M, Schneider M, Buadze A, Gehring M-T, Dube A, Caflisch C. High-dose benzodiazepine dependence: A qualitative study of patients' perceptions on initiation, reasons for use, and obtainment. PLoS One. 2015;**10**:e0142057

[46] Ashton H. Benzodiazepines: How They Work & How to Withdraw. Available from: https://benzo.org.uk/manual/index.htm [Accessed: February 23, 2018]

[47] Ashton H. The Treatment of Benzodiazepine Dependence. Available from: https://benzo.org.uk/ashtbd.htm [Accessed: February 23, 2018]

[48] Clinical Guidelines for Withdrawal Management and Treatment of Drug Dependence in Closed Settings. WHO Guidelines Approved by the Guidelines Review Committee. Geneva: World Health Organization; 2009

[49] World Benzodiazepine Awareness Day. Available from: http://w-bad.org. [Accessed: February 25, 2018]

Section 3

Pharmacokinetic of Drugs, Effect of Compound Interactions on Cytochrome P450 Activity

Clinical Pharmacokinetics of Clavulanic Acid, a Novel β-Lactamase Isolated from *Streptomyces clavuligerus* and Its Variability

Anab Fatima, Mohammad Jiyad Shaikh, Hina Zahid,
Ishart Younus, Sheikh Abdul Khaliq and
Farah Khalid

Additional information is available at the end of the chapter

http://dx.doi.org/10.5772/intechopen.79409

Abstract

The clavulanic acid derived by fermentation of *Streptomyces clavuligerus* and possessed the capability to inactivate a broad range of β-lactamase enzymes. A complex physico-chemical process involves the binding of clavulanic acid to β-lactamases in which clavulanic acid itself deplete irreversibly along with β-lactamase enzyme rendering amoxicillin spared which otherwise would hydrolyze by an enzyme. It is therefore termed as 'suicide 'inhibitor for β-lactamases. We discussed here pharmacokinetic parameters and identified factors responsible for the variability of absorption of clavulanic acid. The results based on individual plasma concentration-time curve of amoxicillin and clavulanic acid in an open, randomized, two-way crossover study involving 10 healthy male subjects administered with two amoxiclav formulations.

Keywords: clinical, clavulanic acid, pharmacokinetics, variable absorption, AUC total, pharmacokinetics, β-lactamase

1. Introduction

Clavulanic acid derived by fermentation of *Streptomyces clavuligerus* and possessed the capability to inactivate a broad range of β-lactamase enzymes. The molecular formula of clavulanate potassium is $C_8H_8KNO_5$ with the molecular weight of 237.25. Chemically it is potassium

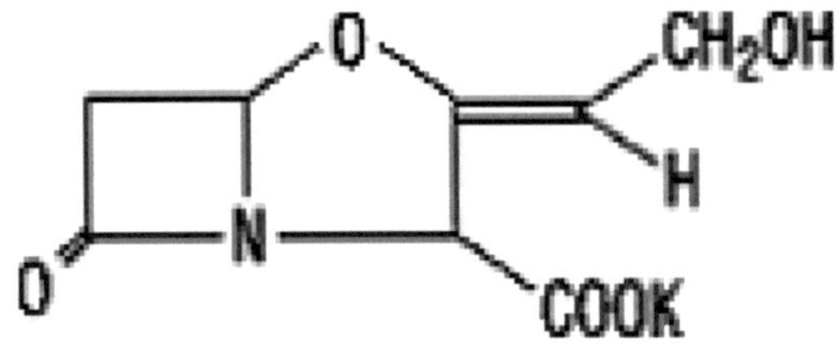

Figure 1. Structure of clavulanate potassium.

(Z)-(2R,5R)-3-(2-hydroxyethylidine)-7-oxo-4-1-azabicyclo[3.2.0]-heptane-2-carboxylate, represented as in **Figure 1**. Mainly it combines with amoxicillin to broaden its antibacterial spectrum [1]. A complex physicochemical process involve in binding of clavulanic acid to β-lactamases in which clavulanic acid itself deplete irreversibly along with β-lactamase enzyme rendering amoxicillin spared which otherwise would hydrolyzed by enzyme. It is therefore termed as 'suicide 'inhibitor for β-lactamases. A very low plasma concentration of clavulanic acid is required for this target action. After oral administration the pharmacokinetic parameters of both components i.e. amoxicillin and clavulanic acid were similar and they did not affect pharmacokinetic parameters of each other [2–6]. This could be one of reason for their antimicrobial combination. In combination clavulanic acid and amoxicillin used in different composition i.e. 250/125, 500/125 and 850/125 respectively. In this amount of amoxicillin varies but that of clavulanic acid remain constant i.e. 125 mg. It would suggest that there is no significant amount required for clavulanic acid to inhibit β lactamase enzymes [3]. We discussed here pharmacokinetic parameters and identified factors responsible for variability of absorption of clavulanic acid and compared it with previous reported data. The results based on individual plasma concentration-time curve of amoxicillin and clavulanic acid in an open, randomized, two-way crossover study involving 12 healthy male subjects administered with two amoxiclav formulations.

2. Parameter which is associated to show variability of absorption

Mainly C_t (concentration at time t) is responsible for clinical effects of any drug. When C_t is higher the AUC (Area under Curve) and C_p (plasma concentration) will also show higher values. Thus they all are co-related to show any clinical effect but question arises that which pharmacokinetic parameter or any other factor is most likely to show variability in absorption of any drug which would ultimately affect its clinical effect. Clavulanic acid along with amoxicillin is well absorbed from stomach after oral administration without having any impact of fasting and fed state on the pharmacokinetics of amoxicillin. While relative bioavailability of clavulanic acid becomes reduced when administered after 30 and 150 min of high fat breakfast. The logic behind reduced bioavailability of clavulanic acid after ingestion with the meal was due to prolong residence time of clavulanic acid in GI due to intragastric tablet deposition in the proximal stomach. The half-life of clavulanic acid is 1.0 h and 25–40% of it is excreted unchanged in urine following first 6 h of administration. Clavulanic acid is difficult to extract out from plasma as it has been bound approximately 25% to human serum and therefore required double extraction procedure to observe by liquid chromatography. After absorption clavulanic acid is well distributed in body tissues [7].

2.1. Content assay for co-amoxiclav tablets by HPLC

The content assay for co-amoxiclav tablets was carried out by validated HPLC method. The method validation was carried out according to USP guidelines. For good and accurate resolution and reproducibility of the presented method various suitability considerations including tailing factor, retention time, resolution, RSD% of retention time and peak areas were determined and were found within acceptable range. The method was found to be specific for the determination of particular analyte. Specificity was determined by injecting the analytical placebo(containing all excipient of tablet except amoxicillin and clavulanic acid). The interference by these excipients were determined by evaluating mixture of all excipient(placebo),standard solutions and commercial pharmaceutical preparations contained amoxicillin and clavulanic acid within the same chromatographic condition.

The linearity of HPLC method was determined for amoxicillin and clavulanic acid. Ten dilutions of amoxicillin and eight dilutions clavulanic acid of different concentrations were prepared in mobile phase then sample size of 20 μl of each concentration was injected into HPLC. The detector response was measured at 235 nm and the calibration plots(concentration versus peak area) were obtained using the linear regression method. The linearity data showed linearity over a concentration range of 0.03–31.25 μg/ml for amoxicillin and 0.24–15.6 μg/ml for clavulanic acid. Repeatable and intermediate precision of method was determined. During the same day with the same experimental condition repeatability of four determination (n = 4) at the same concentration was calculated. The results of assay were compared and evaluated on three different days by different analyst for intermediate precision. The precision values for amoxicillin and clavulanic acid were found to be 0.91 and 0.35% for intraday and 0.89 and 0.34% for inter-day respectively.

The recovery studies were carried out for the assurance of reliability and accuracy of the proposed method. A known quantity of the drug added with preanalyzed sample and then reanalyzed by the proposed method. The recovery studies for amoxicillin and clavulanic acid were performed at three different concentrations corresponded to 80, 100 and 120% of active ingredients. For each concentration mean %recovery were from 99.7 to 101.4 for amoxicillin and 100 to 101.4% for clavulanic acid.

Small variation in the method parameters was created to measure its reliability during routine usage and the robustness. Not any significant effect on the method performance was observed by changing the flow rate of mobile phase, column temperature and ratio of organic content in mobile phase indicated that the test method was robust for all variable conditions (**Table 1**).

2.2. Pharmacokinetic evaluation of co-amoxiclav tablet

In Pakistan Co-amoxiclav tablet of 375 mg marketed by a multinational company Code #1 Pakistan and a local company Code #2 (**Table 2**). Physico-chemical and potency determination

Medium	Parameters	Amoxicillin	Clavulanic acid
In mobile phase/plasma	Limit of Quantification {LOQ(μg/ml)}	0.030/0.0075	0.243/0.12
	Limit of Detection {LOD(μg/ml)}	0.015/0.0037	0.12/0.06

Table 1. Validation parameters of amoxicillin and clavulanic acid in mobile phase.

Name of product	Strength (mg)	Date of mfg.	Date of exp.	Retail price (Rs)	Industrial supplier
(AMCL1)	250/125	02–12	08–13	75.00	Code#1
(AMCL2)	250/125	04–12	04–14	82.00	Code#2

Note: This was a 2 year study and during this period we have taken products from different lots available in the market.

Table 2. Details of different amoxicillin/clavulanic acid products available in Pakistan.

from both sources of different batch were analyzed. This analysis was carried out just to compare the two different brands available in Pakistan as an added parameter. The main objective of study is to conduct pharmacokinetic study of Co-amoxiclav tablet from a multinational company in local population and to find out difference in the pharmacokinetic parameters with the previous reported data due to racial inconsistency. It was preferred to compare only multinational brand because this has been most commonly prescribed by the prescriber to treat infections and the local brand did not proved to be as efficacious as that of multinational brand.

The study was two treatments, two sequences, single dose and cross over design in 12 normal healthy volunteers. An equal number of volunteers were assigned to each sequence. The study covers to determine the pharmacokinetic parameters i.e. Cmax, Tmax, AUC, rate constant, Vd, total clearance and T½ of Co-amoxiclav in local population. The subjects engaged in the study were member of community at large and full-fill all of criteria to be included in the study. This criterion includes healthy males with normal vital signs, blood hematology and chemistry, non-smoker, able to consent and swallow. The study design was endorsed by the National Bioethics Committee, Ministry of Health, Government of Pakistan, Islamabad after critical ethical review and a written informed duly signed by volunteers has been taken. Four volunteers withdraw during study.

2.3. Bioanalytical validation

Plasma amoxicillin and clavulanic acid concentrations were determined using validated methods such as LC/MS/MS analysis (GTF) [8] (**Table 3**). The method was also validated according to International Council for Harmonization (ICH) guidelines (**Figures 2** and **3**).

The fundamental parameters of validation were Specificity, linearity, accuracy, precision, sensitivity, reproducibility, stability and robustness. All these parameters were determined and validated.

Product name	% labeled strength	Product name	% labeled strength
AMCL1	106.1	CODE #1	113.38
AMCL2	119.8	CODE #2	109.9
Mean	112.9		111.64
S.D	9.6		2.46

>> Amoxicillin and clavulanate potassium tablets contain equivalent of not less than 90.0% and not more than 120.0% of the labeled amount of amoxicillin and clavulanic acid (USP 28).

Table 3. HPLC assay of different brands of amoxicillin/clavulanic acid tablet (250/125 mg) available in Pakistan.

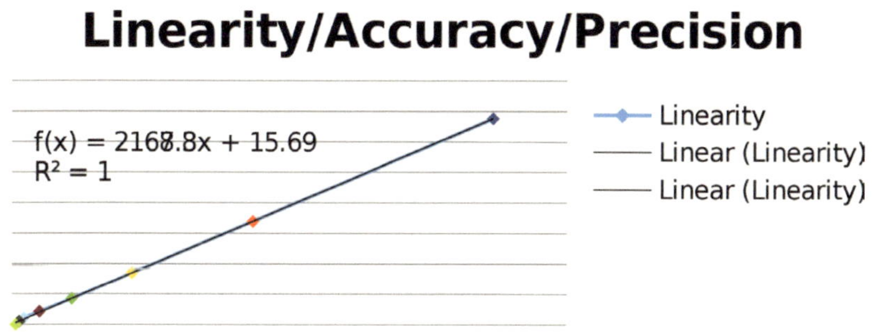

Figure 2. Linearity curve of clavulanic acid: conc vs. area showing linearity between standard solution and peak area.

Mobile Phase containing methanol (10 volume) and 0.02 M disodium hydrogen phosphate buffer (90 volume). The pH was adjusted to 3.0 by phosphoric acid. The mobile phase was filtered and degassed. An HPLC isocratic pump with UV–VIS detector was attached with RP 18e column (Hibar, 250 × 4.6 cm).

In a glass stoppered 15 ml centrifuge tube 0.75 ml of acetonitrile was added to 0.5 ml of plasma. After mixing(30s) the mixture centrifuged for 10 min at 5000 × g. Then 2.5 ml of dichloromethane was added to 300 μl of supernatant. After mixing (30 s) the mixture centrifuge for 10 min at 5000 × g. Then 20 μl of supernatant was injected into liquid chromatograph at 235 nm detection wave length.

2.4. Pattern of variable absorption of clavulanic acid from different oral formulations of co-amoxiclav in healthy subjects

There has been no study to compare the difference of blood concentration time curve of different formulations of co-amoxiclav in local population of Pakistan. Therefore author tried to focus on the Pharmacokinetic pattern especially of clavulanic acid. It is due to fact that absorption of clavulanic acid, after oral administration, is highly variable and may vary over a five-fold range between patients [9]. Based on the plasma amoxicillin and clavulanic acid concentrations of individual subjects, were calculated by applying both compartmental and non-compartmental method of analysis. As best fitted pharmacokinetic model one compartmental

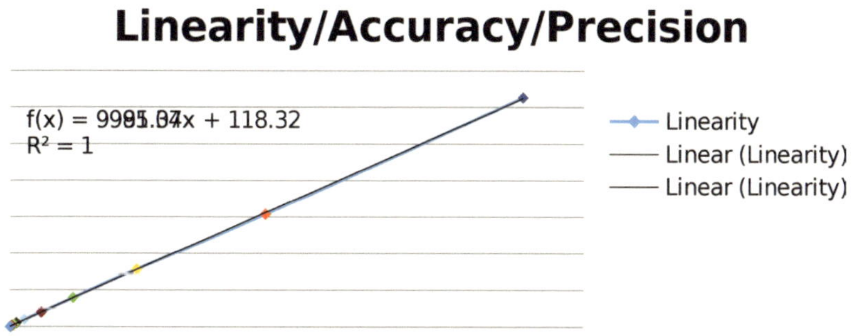

Figure 3. Linearity curve of amoxicillin: conc vs. area showing linearity between standard solution and peak area.

model with lag time, first order absorption and first order elimination was selected for both amoxicillin and clavulanate potassium.

The software Kinetica™ Ver 4.4.1. (Thermo Electron Corporation, USA) used to determine all parameters including both compartmental and non-compartmental analysis and interrelated for any variation in AUCt and demographic facts. The parameters determined were:

Cmax, Tmax (observed and calculated), Ka, Kel, T½ ka, T½α. AUC*0−t*, AUC*0−α*, ƛz, Vz, Vss, AUC last. AUC extrapolated, AUC total, %AUC extrapolated, AUMC and MRT.

where Cmax is maximum plasma concentration of drug(mg/L), Tmax is time required to achieve Cmax(h), Ka is absorption rate constant, AUC0−t, AUC0−α, AUC last with the help of linear trapezoidal method to find area under plasma-concentration time curve up to last measurable concentration (mg.h./L),Kel is elimination half-life (h), ƛz is terminal rate constant, Vz is apparent volume of distribution during terminal phase (L/kg), Vss is apparent volume of distribution at steady state (L/kg), AUMC is area under the first moment of concentration-time curve from time zero to infinity (amount.(time)^2/volume) and MRT is mean residence time (h).

The mean ± plasma concentration time-curve of co-amoxiclav (250/125 mg) tablet of formulation 1 is shown in **Figure 4** in healthy volunteers (n = 8). The other formulation showed similar results. The half-life of all both formulation was 1.34 ± 0.06 h for amoxicillin and 1.20 ± 0.03 h for clavulanic acid.

The area under the concentration-time curve of clavulanic acid is the best measure of the absorption and beneficial effects in the recipient. Calculating the area under the curve using trough and peak blood levels versus using isolated readings for either of these levels alone is the most effective method of monitoring.

The mean AUC0−α values calculated through compartmental analysis were 26.81 ± 0.70 μg.h/ml for amoxicillin while for clavulanate potassium 7.90 ± 0.13 μg.h/ml. The values of mean AUClast and AUCtot from non-compartmental analysis were 23.33 ± 0.70 and 27.96 ± 0.76 μg.h/ml for amoxicillin. The clavulanate potassium showed the values of AUC last and AUC tot were 7.05 ± 0.11 and 7.70 ± 0.16 μg.h/ml.

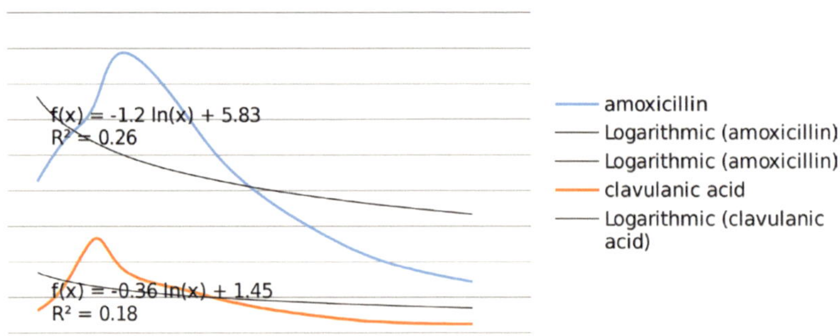

Figure 4. Comparison of mean (±S.D) plasma-concentration time profile of amoxicillin and clavulanic acid after oral dose of 250/125 mg co-amoxiclav tablet (n-8: Formulation 1).

The maximum concentration Cmax of amoxicillin was achieved in 1.85 ± 0.01 h for amoxicillin in compartmental. Similarly Cmax for clavulanate potassium was achieved in 1.56 ± 0.01 h in compartmental analysis (**Tables 4** and **5**).

The reported values of Vss after IV administration for amoxicillin is 0.28 ± 0.06 L/kg, and the Vss of clavulanic acid as 0.24 ± 0.06 L/kg, showing ratio for the volume of distribution between clavulanic acid and amoxicillin as 0.8571 [14] and therefore on the basis of this the ratio of amoxicillin to clavulanic acid AUCs should be 3.4, when co-amoxiclav is at dose of 250/125. The author observed in this study, the lowest AUCt amoxicillin/clavulanic acid ratio was 2.7 ± 0.50 at the lower doses used. This would assume equal absorption of both amoxicillin and clavulanic acid. But in the same dose amoxicillin/clavulanic acid AUCt ratios was higher that would suggest that with a similar amoxicillin absorption, clavulanic acid absorption must have been reduced. The reported absolute bioavailability of clavulanic acid, when co-administered with amoxicillin has been ranged from 31.4 to 98.8% [10]. Further it is reported that there is no major alteration in the mean AUCt of 125 mg clavulanate when it is administered along 500 mg of amoxicillin, but it creates marked impact on the coefficient of variation for the AUC which alter from 27.6% for clavulanic acid alone to 45.6% when given with amoxicillin [15]. Various other studies showed mean absorption up to 97% when clavulanic acid administered alone with minor inter-patient variability. It indicates interaction between absorption of amoxicillin and clavulanic acid [11, 12] . The author further found that there was no significant variation in the AUC observed for amoxicillin in this study either among subjects, on the basis of demographic data, or between formulations, once corrected for the dose. On the contrary, high variability was seen between subjects in the AUC of clavulanic acid (**Figure 5**). There were all healthy male subjects (with normal renal function), and it is difficult to explain the high variability seen in the clavulanic acid AUC on patient factors. However, it has been reported in other studies [13]. Also study observed broadened Tmax i.e. increase lag time indicating a rate limiting step in the absorption process. The authors being able to show that two different co-amoxiclav formulations each gave a variation in the absorption, or in the AUCt value, of clavulanic acid for the same 125 mg dose.

In a study reported broadened Tmax with high dose of amoxicillin (875 mg) indicate a rate limiting step in the absorption and support previous other studies [16].

In this study the authors tried to show variation in the absorption or in AUCt value of clavulanic acid at 125 mg dose with two formulations. Although we did not find any report of therapy failure among the patients due to this variation and its clinical efficacy has been maintained. It would suggest that it is more important to focus on the absolute or fixed amount of clavulanic acid rather than on its plasma concentration.

Formulation	**Dose (mg)**	**$T_{1/2}$ (h)**	**T_{max} (h)**	**C_{max} (μg/L)**	**AUC (μg.h/L)**
AMCL1	125	1.20 ± 0.02	1.56 ± 0.01	2.60 ± 0.03	8.30 ± 0.06
AMCL2	125	1.21 ± 0.03	1.54 ± 0.02	1.98 ± 0.70	7.90 ± 0.13

Table 4. Pharmacokinetic parameters of clavulanic acid.

Formulation	Dose (mg)	$T_{1/2}$ (h)	T_{max} (h)	C_{max} (μg/L)	AUC (μg.h/L)
AMCL1	250	1.34 ± 0.06	1.85 ± 0.01	2.98 ± 0.27	26.81 ± 0.70
AMCL2	250	1.32 ± 0.05	1.83 ± 0.02	3.3 ± 1.12	26.98 ± 0.83

Table 5. Pharmacokinetic parameters of amoxicillin.

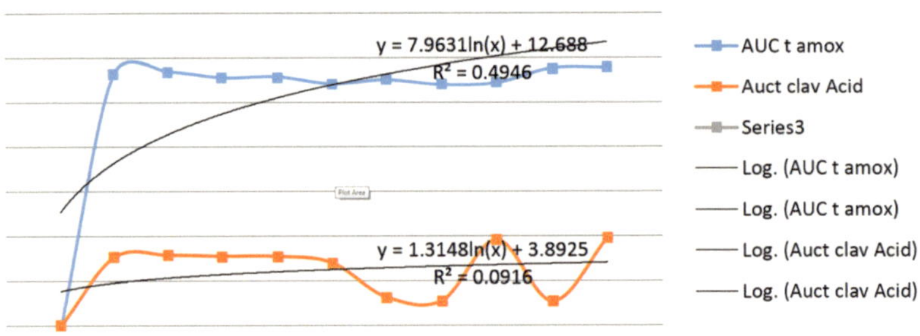

Figure 5. Individual AUCts of amoxicillin plotted versus the AUCts of clavulanic acid. It can be seen that there is a variation in the AUCts of clavulanic acid, with little variation in those of amoxicillin (95% confidence interval).

3. Conclusions

In conclusion, variable absorption nature of clavulanic acid has been highlighted with alteration in AUCt ratio of co-amoxiclav without any known cause. However, it is evident from clinical data that there is not any variability in the efficacy of co-amoxiclav and that the current dosage ratio of 4:1 holds a traditional value.

The study requires further evaluation to find out the reason for this variation.

Acknowledgements

The authors are thankful to National Bioethics committee, Ministry of Health, Islamabad, Pakistan, for expert ethical review and guidance. Also humble co-operation from administrative and Paramedic staff of Imam Clinic Hospital Karachi and from all volunteers is highly acknowledged.

Conflict of interest

There is no actual or potential conflict of interest between authors relative to this activity including financial relationship.

Author details

Anab Fatima[1]*, Mohammad Jiyad Shaikh[2], Hina Zahid[1], Ishart Younus[3], Sheikh Abdul Khaliq[3] and Farah Khalid[1]

*Address all correspondence to: anabfatima@gmail.com

1 Faculty of Pharmacy, Dow University of Health Sciences, Karachi, Pakistan

2 Unilever Karachi, Pakistan

3 Faculty of Pharmacy, Hamdard University, Karachi, Pakistan

References

[1] Cooper CE, Slocombe B, White AR. Effect of low concentrations of clavulanic acid on the invitro activity of amoxycillin against β-lactamase producing *Branhamella catharrhasis* and *Haemophilus influenzae*. The Journal of Antimicrobial Chemotherapy. 1990;**6**:371-380

[2] Adam D, de Visser I, Koeppe P. Pharmacokinetics of amoxicillin andclavulanic acid administered alone and in combination. Antimicrobial Agents and Chemotherapy. 1982;**22**:353-357

[3] Reed MD. The clinical pharmacology of amoxicillin and clavulanic acid. Pediatric Infectious Disease Journal. 1998;**17**:957-962

[4] Soback S, Bor A, Kurtz B, Paz R, Ziv G. Clavulanate-potentiated amoxycillin: in vitro antibacterial activity and oral bioavailability in calves. Journal of Veterinary Pharmacology and Therapeutics. 1987;**10**:105-113

[5] Todd PA, Benfield P. Amoxicillin/clavulanic acid: An update of its antibacterial activity, pharmacokinetic properties and therapeutic use. Drugs. 1990;**39**:264-307

[6] Vogelmann B, Gudmundsson S, Leggett J, Turnidge J, Ebert S, Craig WA. Correlation of antimicrobial pharmacokinetic parameters with therapeutically efficacy in an animal model. The Journal of Infectious Diseases. 1998;**158**:831-847

[7] Weitschies W, Friedrich C, Wedemeyer RS, Schmidtmann M, et al. Bioavailability of amoxicillin and clavulanic acid from extended release tablets depends on intragastric tablet deposition and gastric emptying. European Journal of Pharmaceutics and Biopharmaceutics. 2008;**70**(2):641-648

[8] Seyed Mohsen Foroutan, AfshinZarghi, Alireza Shafaati, Arash Khoddam et al.Simultaneous determination of amoxicillin and clavulanic acid in human plasma by isocratic reversed-phase HPLC using UV detection, Journal of Pharmaceutical and Biomedical Analysis. 2007;**45**(3):531-534

[9] Vree TB, Dammers E, Exler PS. Identical pattern of highly variable absorption of clavulanic acid from four different oral formulations of co-amoxiclav in healthy subjects. The Journal of Antimicrobial Chemotherapy. 2003;**51**(2):373-378

[10] Nilsson-Ehle I, Fellner H, Hedström SA, Nilsson-Ehle P, Sjövall J. Pharmacokinetics of clavulanic acid, given in combination with amoxicillin, in volunteers. Journal of Antimicrobial Chemotherapy. 1985;**16**:491-496

[11] Allen GD, Coates PE, Davies BE. On the absorption of clavulanic acid. Biopharmaceutics and Drug Disposition. 1988;**9**:127-136

[12] Bolton GC, Allen GD, Davies BE, Filer CW, Jeffery DJ. The disposition of clavulanic acid in man. Xenobiotica. 1986;**16**:853-863

[13] Elias Jones A, Barnes ND, Tasker TCG, Horton R. Pharmacokinetics of intravenous amo xycillin and potassium clavulanate in seriously ill children. Journal of Antimicrobial Chemotherapy. 1990;**25**:269-274

[14] Horber FF, Frey FJ, Descoeurders C, Murray AT, Reubi FC. Differential effect of impaired renal function on the kinetics of clavulanic acid and amoxicillin. Antimicrobial Agents and Chemotherapy. 1986;**29**:614-619

[15] Witkowski G, Lode H, Höffken G, Koeppe P. Pharmacokinetic studies of amoxicillin, potassium clavulanate and their combination. European Journal of Clinical Microbiology. 1982;**1**:233-237

[16] Chulavatnatol S, Charles BG. Determination of dose-dependent absorption of amoxycillin from urinary excretion data in healthy subjects. British Journal of Clinical Pharmacology. 1994;**38**:274-277

Chapter 7

New Antituberculosis Drug FS-1

Rinat Islamov, Bahkytzhan Kerimzhanova and Alexander Ilin

Additional information is available at the end of the chapter

http://dx.doi.org/10.5772/intechopen.80795

Abstract

The new iodine complex (FS-1), including molecular iodine, which is coordinated by lithium, magnesium halides, and bioorganic ligands, possesses high bactericidal activity against various microorganisms, including *Mycobacterium* sp., *Staphylococcus aureus* MRSA and MSSA, *Escherichia coli, Pseudomonas aeruginosa,* etc. FS-1 has synergistic properties with a broad class of antibiotics. The experimental model of tuberculosis in guinea pigs caused by clinical multidrug-resistant strains of *Mycobacterium tuberculosis* shows antituberculosis, immunomodulatory, and anti-inflammatory activity. FS-1 is characterized by low acute toxicity and lack of genotoxicity and mutagenicity. FS-1 is well distributed to organs and tissues; its pharmacokinetics is linear. The maximum nontoxic dose is 100 mg/kg for rats after 28-day oral administration and 30 mg/kg for rabbits after 180-day oral administration.

Keywords: *Mycobacterium tuberculosis*, iodine, complex, antimicrobial activity, antimicrobial resistance, tuberculosis, antituberculosis drug, preclinical trials, toxicity

1. Introduction

Antimicrobial resistance (AMR) has long been recognized as a global problem [1, 2]. At that, the solution to this problem is complicated by the fact that as soon as a new antibiotic appears, it is immediately reported about resistance to it. For example, some isolates of *Pseudomonas aeruginosa* and *Burkholderia cenocepacia* showed intermediate resistance to a new antibiotic eravacycline as early as at the stage of clinical trials, although the antibiotic effectiveness is very high against other bacteria, including the multiresistant ones [3]. Sometimes this resistance can be natural, for example, to pyrazinamide in *Mycobacterium bovis* [4, 5]. A widely practiced method of reducing AMR, the cyclic and mixed use of antibiotics that belong to alternative classes, has proved to be ineffective [6].

Pulmonary tuberculosis poses a particular problem. The global WHO report announced the number of new tuberculosis cases detected in 2015—2110.4 million, of which 480,000 new cases of multidrug-resistant tuberculosis (MDR-TB) and 7579 cases of extensively drug-resistant TB (XDR-TB). The greatest number of the disease cases is registered in six countries—India, Indonesia, China, Nigeria, Pakistan, and South Africa—60% of the worldwide incidence [7]. Despite the emergence of new antituberculosis drugs, the situation with high resistance of *M. tuberculosis* remains difficult [7, 8]. In this regard, the search and development of new anti-infectious drugs are extremely relevant.

Among the numerous substances with high antimicrobial activity, resistance to which was not detected or it remains at the minimum level, there are polymeric complexes of iodine [9, 10]. Iodine complexes have broad antimicrobial, anti-inflammatory, immunomodulatory, and antitumor activity [11–16]. Really interesting are nanocomposites with molecular iodine, which are superior in their antimicrobial activity to the widely known complex of polyvinylpyrrolidone and iodine (PVP-iodine) [17, 18]. The ability of molecular iodine to form complexes with a variety of properties and compositions with ligands of different nature makes it very promising to develop drugs based on iodine coordination compounds [19–24].

The new drug FS-1 relates to iodine coordination compounds with bioorganic ligands, magnesium, and lithium cations. The active center of FS-1 included α-dextrin helix with molecular iodine (I_2) that is coordinated with lithium halogenides and amide groups of protein component. Such a structure protects I_2 from interaction with bioorganic compounds after oral intake. Bioorganic compounds are only able to compete with I_2 in complexing if donor activity is greater as against amide groups [24–26].

The developed drug FS-1 possesses broad antimicrobial activity against antibiotic-resistant and antibiotic-susceptible Gram-positive and Gram-negative bacteria, mycobacteria, fungi, and viruses [27–33].

Both liquid and solid dosage forms of FS-1 were produced from the pharmaceutical development process [34]. Preclinical trials of the drug FS-1 were conducted according to the recommendations of the International Conference on Harmonization of Technical Requirements for Registration of Pharmaceuticals for Human Use (ICH). This chapter will present the major results from preclinical trials of the new drug FS-1, conducted in 2004–2014.

2. In vitro antimicrobial activity

The aim of these studies presented here was to assess the in vitro antimicrobial activity of FS-1. By using a serial dilution technique assay, the activities of FS-1 were tested against both on typified bacteria and on clinical isolates. **Table 1** shows a list of microorganisms that were used to examine the in vitro effectiveness of FS-1 [27–29, 33, 35, 36].

The minimum inhibitory concentration (MIC) was in the range of 0.02–0.3 mg/mL. At the same time, clinical isolates *M. tuberculosis* SCAID 187.0 (MDR); 562, 892, 535, and 722

Typified bacteria	Clinical isolates
M. tuberculosis H37Rv*	*M. tuberculosis* MS-115 (MDR), SCAID 187.0 (MDR); 562, 892, 535, and 722* (isoniazid-resistant); *M. bovis*** 2, 3, and 5; *M. avium* 780
	*Yersinia pestis****, *Bacillus anthracis****, *Brucella* sp.***
Staphylococcus aureus ATCC 6538-P B-RKM 0039, *S. aureus* ATCC 29213—oxacillin-susceptible strain (MSSA), *S. aureus* ATCC 43300—methicillin- and oxacillin-resistant (MRSA), *S. aureus* ATCC 29213, *S. aureus* ATCC 43300, *Escherichia coli* ATCC 25922, and ATCC BAA-196 and *Candida albicans* ATCC 18814	*S. aureus*****—114 MRSA and MSSA clinical isolates—*P. aeruginosa* № 4/32, *E. coli* O55 № 12, *C. albicans* 3/4

*Collections of microorganisms at the National Scientific Center for Pulmonology, Kazakhstan.
**At Kazakh Scientific Research Veterinary Institute.
***At Kazakh Scientific Center for Quarantine and Zoonotic Diseases.
****At Institute of Experimental Pathology and Parasitology, Bulgaria.

Table 1. List of bacteria and their characteristics used to examine antimicrobial activity of FS-1.

(isoniazid-resistant); and *M. bovis* 2, 3, and 5 showed the greatest susceptibility [36]. The MIC of FS-1 against *Y. pestis* and *B. anthracis* was 0.2 mg/mL [35].

FS-1 causes lysis of the bacterial cell, damaging the cell membrane [37]. A study on the membrane lytic activity of FS-1 on *M. smegmatis* by electron microscopy showed that the bacterial cell lysis occurs within 5–30 minutes at a concentration of FS-1 of 4 μg/mL. In addition, FS-1 inhibits DNA-dependent RNA polymerase (RNAP) of *M. tuberculosis* forming a complex between bacterial DNA and magnesium ion in RNAP [26].

Most bacterial diseases including tuberculosis are treated with a combination of multiple drugs in a regimen. Synergistic effects with existing drugs are valuable characteristics of a new drug candidate. FS-1 was tested in combination with antibiotics and various first and second antituberculosis drugs (ATBD). Synergy between drugs and FS-1 was determined by chequerboard in vitro [27]. Testing showed that synergy between FS-1 and antituberculosis drugs (ATBD) was observed against both on susceptibility and on multidrug resistance MTB. Among the cephalosporins, only cefamandole showed synergy with FS-1 against clinical isolates *S. aureus*. The index of fractional inhibitory concentration was 0.62 [27]. Thus, according to the results of testing, in vitro the FS-1 is an effective compound of a class of iodine coordination compounds.

3. In vivo antituberculosis activity

The most important stage of preclinical studies of new drugs is the evaluation of efficacy in animal models. There are various animal *M. tuberculosis* infection models. The most common are guinea pigs and mice. A classical guinea pig model of tuberculosis caused by highly virulent clinical strains of *M. tuberculosis* MS-115 and SCAID 187.0 isolated from patients with MDR-TB was used in the study on the therapeutic effectiveness of FS-1 [8, 29, 38].

The efficacy result of the tuberculosis model showed that the FS-1 combination regimen reduced the bacterial load in comparison with standard therapy. A primary characteristic of the therapeutic activity of FS-1 was an increase in the effectiveness when combined with ATBD including isoniazid, rifampicin, pyrazinamide, cycloserine, protionamide, capreomycin, and amikacin [29, 30]. It was noted that in the treatment of tuberculosis in guinea pigs with FS-1 *M. tuberculosis* acquired susceptibility to first-line ATBD. Apparently this is due to the effect of FS-1 on the *M. tuberculosis* genome [30]. In the studies on other bacteria, *Streptococcus mutans* and *S. aureus* and *S. epidermidis*, iodine complexes have been shown to influence the transcription activity in microbial genome [39–41].

The therapeutic effect on the guinea pig body has also been noted. In particular, the exposure to FS-1 inhibits the development of inflammation in tuberculosis and increases the airiness of the lung parenchyma and permeability of capillaries [29]. This is due to the ability of iodine complexes to inhibit the production of NO and TNF-alpha and increase mucociliary clearance in the respiratory tract [15, 42]. In addition, combination therapy with FS-1 and ATBD reduces the incidence of adverse reactions and toxic effects of the drugs in animals [30].

In the studies presented here, the combination of FS-1 in MDR-TB animal models is significantly more effective than therapy only with ATBD.

4. Toxicity studies

The toxicity of FS-1 was examined in both liquid form and tablets [34, 43].

The median cytotoxic concentration (CC_{50}) of FS-1 on the MDCK cells exceeds 5 mg/mL [44]. In vitro and in vivo genotoxicity and mutagenic potential of FS-1 were examined in mice with Ames test, micronucleus, and comet assays. According to the results from the studies, FS-1 does not induce gene mutations or chromosomal abnormalities [45, 46].

Acute toxicity study of FS-1 liquid dosage form was carried out after intravenous administration to rodents, mice (CD-1), and rats (Wistar) [47]. The median lethal dose (LD_{50}) was 65 mg/kg in mice and 100 mg/kg in rats. After the administration of FS-1, the following signs were observed in animals: exophthalmos, piloerection, impaired motor coordination, paroxysmal convulsions of lower limbs, bradycardia, and tachypnea. Death occurred within 24 hours after the administration of FS-1. Necropsy revealed a disturbance of blood circulation in the heart, liver, and kidneys and pulmonary edema in dead animals. Microscopic examination showed plethora and inflammatory infiltration in the lungs, liver, and kidneys and diapedesis hemorrhages in the myocardium. At the same time, there were no changes in the thyroid gland [47].

After oral administration of FS-1 liquid form to rats (Wistar), LD_{50} was not achieved. The maximum administered dose of FS-1 was 466 mg/kg. The minimal dose of FS-1 did not cause damage to the mucous membrane of the gastrointestinal tract (GIT). Medium and high doses provoked minimal damage to the gastric mucosa. Histological examination of thyroid gland did not reveal the pathological changes [47].

Toxicokinetics (TK) of FS-1 liquid form was examined in male and female rats after single oral administration at doses of 233, 116, and 30 mg/kg [48]. The content of FS-1 was measured in the blood, heart, lungs, liver, kidneys, and spleen. The primary TK parameters were calculated by non-compartmental method. The maximum concentration of FS-1 in the blood (C_{max}) and the time it was reached (t_{max}) were found visually on the graph. The TK parameters for oral doses of FS-1 are given in **Table 2**.

FS-1 is absorbed quite rapidly from the gastrointestinal tract; the maximum values of its concentrations in the blood were reached within 1–1.5 hours after its administration. During the first 10–30 minutes, the concentration of FS-1 in the blood increased and reached a maximum after 2 hours. The level of the drug was further reduced, and at the end of 96 hours, the detection limit was reached. High values of the volume of distribution, according to the generally accepted point of view, can be interpreted as a sign of a wide distribution of the drug in the body. At the same time, the rate of distribution of FS-1 in the organs was lower than in the blood, therefore, accumulation does not take place. The nature of the relationship between the dose of FS-1 and the area under the pharmacokinetic curve (AUC) in the blood, as well as the constancy of the invariant TK parameters, indicate that the dynamics of drug absorption, distribution, and elimination obey the basic principles of linear kinetics. The primary metabolites of FS-1 include iodides, which are excreted in the urine [48].

In addition, chronic toxicity was examined during 180-day oral administration in rabbits. The characteristic symptoms of iodine toxicity in rabbits were not detected at a dose of 30 mg/kg [47–51].

Despite the fact that iodine does not have mutagenic properties, there is evidence of the effect of high iodide doses on the development of mice. Although the mechanisms of toxic effect of

TK parameter	**Dose, mg/kg**		
	30	**116**	**233**
AUC(mg·h/L)	138.2 ± 19.5	382.4 ± 49.6	669.5 ± 103.1
Cl (L·h/kg)	0.22 ± 0.03	0.30 ± 0.04	0.35 ± 0.05
MRT (h)	24.6 ± 3.5	20.2 ± 2.7	23.1 ± 3.6
β (h^{-1})	0.026 ± 0.003	0.025 ± 0.004	0.026 ± 0.004
V_β (L/kg)	8.2 ± 1.2	12.0 ± 1.6	13.5 ± 2.1
C_{max} (mg/L)	9.0 ± 0.2	34.1 ± 5.0	45.1 ± 9.6
t_{max} (h)	2	1	1
$t_{1/2(\beta)}$ (h)	26.6 ± 3.7	26.6 ± 3.6	26.6 ± 3.7

Table 2. Toxicokinetic parameters of FS-1 after single oral administration of three doses to rats by non-compartmental method, n = 6.

high iodide doses on pregnant females and embryos have not been revealed, it is assumed that this is due to impaired thyroid function in pregnant females. Thyroid hormones in turn affect sex glands of animals [52]. An evaluation of the embryotoxic properties of FS-1 was performed on a bird model using *Gallus gallus* chicken embryos at different developmental stages [53]. Embryotoxicity was assessed by the effect of FS-1 on survival and developmental pathology. At a concentration of 3 mg/mL, the mortality rate of 10-day embryos was 100%, whereas for 12- and 18-day-old embryos, it was 80 and 50%, respectively. At the same time, developmental abnormalities were not detected. The toxicity of FS-1 toward chicken embryos depends on the concentration and developmental stage [54]. The Spearman's correlation coefficient was greater than 0.976 at $p < 0.001$, which indicates a high dependence. It is known that iodides can exhibit toxicity to the reproductive function in two ways: through oxidative stress in the testis of rats and thyroid dysfunction in pregnant females [52, 55].

One of the problems encountered in the clinical trials of new drugs is that there could be various unforeseen immunotoxic reactions [56, 57]. As already noted, iodine complexes have immunotropic properties [15, 58]. Therefore, the immunotoxicity and allergenicity of FS-1 were studied in various tests:

a. Intradermal and conjunctival test

b. Active and passive (ovary) cutaneous anaphylaxis

c. mast cell degranulation

d. Anaphylactogenicity

e. Induction of delayed-type hypersensitivity reaction

f. Analysis of changes in mass and cellularity of the popliteal lymph node

g. Assessment of specific lysis of human peripheral blood leukocytes

h. Analysis of the relative count of basophils and eosinophils in human peripheral blood

i. Determination of mass and cellularity of immune organs and antibody response in guinea pigs

The study found that FS-1 does not possess anaphylactogenicity, does not cause type I allergic reaction and does not influence the formation of a delayed-type hypersensitivity reaction, does not have immunopathological and immunotoxic effects, and does not cause disorders and/or dysfunctions in the processes involved in normal maintenance of immune status in the tested doses, even against the background of antigenic stimulus [59, 60].

The preparation of a tablet dosage form of FS-1 is the most important stage in the pharmaceutical development of novel drug [34, 61, 62].

After the oral administration of FS-1 tablets to rats (Wistar), LD_{50} was found to exceed 2000 mg/kg [43]. The observed clinical and pathomorphological signs of damage to the body of animals with FS-1 are similar to the symptoms of poisoning with iodine solutions [50].

Toxicology of iodides and iodates was well studied in numerous animal species, as well as in humans, whereas the data on iodine complexes including Lugol's solution and PVP-iodine are very scarce [51, 63].

The toxicity of FS-1 tablets associated with repeated administration was examined in rats (Wistar) after 28-day oral administration. It was found that the organs for the damaging action of FS-1 included the thyroid gland, liver, and kidneys. There were changes in the blood parameters: the levels of leukocytes and lymphocytes and alanine aminotransferase and aspartate aminotransferase increased. But these changes were reversible, and after 28 days of recovery period, all parameters were normalized [43].

It is known that prolonged exposure to or intake of high doses of the iodine-containing drugs is accompanied by thyrotoxic reactions in the form of iodine-induced hypothyroidism [64]. Due to excessive intake of iodine, the Wolff-Chaikoff effect occurs, which develops within a few days [65]. This is accompanied by a temporary reduction of the thyroid hormone level due to a decrease in the Na+/I-symporter activity (NIS) [66]. The Wolff-Chaikoff effect is transient, and the level of hormones with the withdrawal of the iodine-containing drugs is restored in a few days. It was noted that the chronic effect of iodine doses (in Japan, for example, up to several milligrams per day are consumed with food, exceeding the WHO recommended standards (90–200 μg)) frequently does not cause any hypothyroid or thyrotoxic conditions [67]. Therefore, rats were also analyzed for the level of thyroid-stimulating hormone (TSH), thyroxine (T4), and triiodothyronine (T3). The findings of the studies have shown that the levels of TSH, T3, and T4 in the blood serum of rats did not change. It has been established that the T3/T4 ratio in all studied groups was in the range of 0.20–0.50. The absence of significant changes in the T3/T4 ratio in animals of all groups indicates a normal rate of deiodization. As a result, the highest nontoxic dose (NOAEL) of FS-1 was established, which was of 100 mg/kg [43]. Summarizing the results obtained, it can be noted that high doses of FS-1 lead to the development of thyrotoxicosis in rats and not hypothyroidism, as with excessive intake of iodides into the animal organism [51].

5. Conclusion

FS-1 is highly effective against various Gram-positive and Gram-negative bacteria, including those resistant to antibiotics. MIC varied over a wide range from 0.02 to 0.3 mg/mL. At that, FS-1 has a synergistic effect with some antimicrobial agents. The main mechanism of action of FS-1 consists in membrane lytic activity. In addition, the investigational drug affects the gene expression in bacteria. The effectiveness of FS-1 in combination with ATBD of the first- and second-line was examined in the guinea pig models of tuberculosis. FS-1 has pronounced anti-inflammatory and antitoxic effects. The CC_{50} value in MDCK cells is more than 5 mg/mL. This is 16 times higher than the MIC. FS-1 does not have mutagenic and genotoxic properties. The acute oral toxicity of FS-1 in rats is LD_{50} of more than 2000 mg/kg. The extent of FS-1 distribution in the organs is not greater than in the blood. Its kinetics is linear. The primary metabolites include iodides. At the same time, FS-1 possesses embryonic toxicity in chicken embryos but does not lead to developmental abnormalities. FS-1 does not cause allergic reactions and does not possess immunotoxic properties. The liver, kidney, and thyroid gland are the target organs for toxic injuries induced by repeated administration of FS-1. At the same time, thyrotoxicosis develops but not hypothyroidism. NOAEL value is 100 mg/kg of rats after 28-day oral administration and 30 mg/kg in rabbits after 180-day administration.

Conflict of interest

Authors report grants from Ministry of Investments and Development of the Republic of Kazakhstan, during the conduct of the studies.

Author details

Rinat Islamov*, Bahkytzhan Kerimzhanova and Alexander Ilin

*Address all correspondence to: renatislamov@gmail.com

Scientific Center for Anti-Infectious Drugs, Almaty, Kazakhstan

References

[1] Ventola CL. The antibiotic resistance crisis: Part 1: Causes and threats. Pharmacy and Therapeutics. 2015;**40**:277-283

[2] Founou RC, Founou LL, Essack SY. Clinical and economic impact of antibiotic resistance in developing countries: A systematic review and meta-analysis. Butaye P, ed. PLoS One. 2017;**12**:e0189621. DOI: 10.1371/journal.pone.0189621

[3] Sutcliffe JA, O'Brien W, Fyfe C, Grossman TH. Antibacterial activity of eravacycline (TP-434), a novel fluorocycline, against hospital and community pathogens. Antimicrobial Agents and Chemotherapy. 2013;**57**:5548-5558. DOI: 10.1128/AAC.01288-13

[4] Davies J, Davies D. Origins and evolution of antibiotic resistance. Microbiology and Molecular Biology Reviews. 2010;**74**:417-433. DOI: 10.1128/MMBR.00016-10

[5] Scorpio A, Zhang Y. Mutations in pncA, a gene encoding pyrazinamidase/nicotinamidase, cause resistance to the antituberculous drug pyrazinamide in tubercle bacillus. Nature Medicine. 1996;**2**:662-667. DOI: 10.1038/nm0696-662

[6] van Duijn PJ, Verbrugghe W, Jorens PG, Spöhr F, Schedler D, Deja M, et al. The effects of antibiotic cycling and mixing on antibiotic resistance in intensive care units: A cluster-randomised crossover trial. The Lancet Infectious Diseases. 2018;**18**:401-409. DOI: 10.1016/S1473-3099(18)30056-2

[7] Global Tuberculosis Report. 2016. Available from: http://apps.who.int/medicinedocs/documents/s23098en/s23098en.pdf [Accessed: July 13, 2018]

[8] Ilin AI, Kerimzhanova BF, Islamov RA. Anti-tuberculosis (TB) drugs and drug resistance. Reports of the National Academy of Sciences of the Republic of Kazakhstan. 2015;**4**:116-134

[9] Bigliardi PL, Alsagoff SAL, El-Kafrawi HY, Pyon JK, Wa CTC, Villa MA. Povidone iodine in wound healing: A review of current concepts and practices. International Journal of Surgery. 2017;**44**:260-268. DOI: 10.1016/j.ijsu.2017.06.073

[10] Malone M, Johani K, Jensen SO, Gosbell IB, Dickson HG, McLennan S, et al. Effect of cadexomer iodine on the microbial load and diversity of chronic non-healing diabetic foot ulcers complicated by biofilm in vivo. Journal of Antimicrobial Chemotherapy. 2017;**72**:2093-2101. DOI: 10.1093/jac/dkx099

[11] Ignatova M, Markova N, Manolova N, Rashkov I. Antibacterial and antimycotic activity of a cross-linked electrospun poly(vinyl pyrrolidone)-iodine complex and a poly(ethylene oxide)/poly(vinyl pyrrolidone)-iodine complex. Journal of Biomaterials Science. Polymer Edition. 2008;**19**:373-386. DOI: 10.1163/156856208783721056

[12] Tang Y, Xie L, Sai M, Xu N, Ding D. Preparation and antibacterial activity of quaternized chitosan with iodine. Materials Science and Engineering. C, Materials for Biological Applications. 2015;**48**:1-4. DOI: 10.1016/j.msec.2014.11.019

[13] Ito H, Ito T, Hikida M, Yashiro J, Otsuka A, Kida H, et al. Outbreak of highly pathogenic avian influenza in Japan and anti-influenza virus activity of povidone-iodine products. Dermatology. 2006;**212**:115-118. DOI: 10.1159/000089210

[14] Nakao H, Yamazaki M, Tsuboi R, Ogawa H. Mixture of sugar and povidone-iodine stimulates wound healing by activating keratinocytes and fibroblast functions. Archives of Dermatological Research. 2006;**298**:175-182. DOI: 10.1007/s00403-006-0683-z

[15] Beukelman CJ, van den Berg AJ, Hoekstra MJ, Uhl R, Reimer K, Mueller S. Anti-inflammatory properties of a liposomal hydrogel with povidone-iodine (Repithel) for wound healing in vitro. Burns. 2008;**34**:845-855. DOI: 10.1016/j.burns.2007.11.014

[16] Alfaro Y, Delgado G, Cárabez A, Anguiano B, Aceves C. Iodine and doxorubicin, a good combination for mammary cancer treatment: Antineoplastic adjuvancy, chemoresistance inhibition, and cardioprotection. Molecular Cancer. 2013;**12**:45. DOI: 10.1186/1476-4598-12-45

[17] Gao B, Wang Z, Liu Q, Du R. Immobilization of povidone-iodine on surfaces of silica gel particles and bactericidal property. Colloids and Surfaces. B, Biointerfaces. 2010;**79**:446-451. DOI: 10.1016/j.colsurfb.2010.05.007

[18] Some S, Sohn JS, Kim J, Lee SH, Lee SC, Lee J, et al. Graphene-iodine nanocomposites: Highly potent bacterial inhibitors that are bio-compatible with human cells. Scientific Reports. 2016;**6**:20015. DOI: 10.1038/srep20015

[19] Betzel C, Hingerty B, Noltemeyer M, Weber G, Hamilton WSJA. (β-Cyclodextrin)2·KI7·9 H_2O. Spatial fitting of a polyiodide chain to a given matrix. Journal of Inclusion Phenomena. 2004;**1**:181-191. DOI: 10.1007/BF00656821

[20] Küpper FC, Feiters MC, Olofsson B, Kaiho T, Yanagida S, Zimmermann MB, et al. Commemorating two centuries of iodine research: An interdisciplinary overview of current research. Angewandte Chemie (International Ed. in English). 2011;**50**:11598-11620. DOI: 10.1002/anie.201100028

[21] Mahmoud KR, Refat MS, Sharshar T, Adam MA, Manaaa E-SA. Synthesis of amino acid iodine charge transfer complexes in situ methanolic medium: Chemical and physical investing. Journal of Molecular Liquids. **222**:1061-1067. DOI: 10.1016/j.molliq.2016.07.138

[22] Berdibay SB, Paretskaya NA, Sabitov AN, Islamov RA, Tamazyan RA, Tokmoldin SZ, et al. Phenylalanine – Iodine complex and its structure. News of the National Academy of Sciences of the Republic of Kazakhstan Physico-Mathematical Series. 2017;**2**:5-9

[23] Barinov D, Bekesheva K, Ustenova G, Kurmanalieva AR, Kalykova AS, Ilin AI. IR spectroscopic study of substances containing iodine adduct. Research Journal of Pharmaceutical, Biological and Chemical Sciences. 2017;**8**:1599-1604

[24] Yuldasheva GA, Zhidomirov GM, Ilin AI. Effect of α-dextrin nanoparticles on the structure of iodine complexes with polypeptides and alkali metal halogenides, and on the mechanisms of their anti-human immunodeficiency virus and anticancer activity. In: Grumezescu A, editor. Design and Development of New Nanocarriers. Elsevier Inc; 2018. pp. 637-685. DOI: 10.1016/B978-0-12-813627-0.00017-X

[25] Ilin AI, Kulmanov ME. Antibacterial agent for treating infectious diseases of bacterial origin [Patent]. Patent US20140010782; A1-2014-09-01

[26] Ilin A, Kerimzhanova B, Yuldasheva G. Action mechanism of molecular iodine complex with bioorganic ligands, magnesium and lithium halogenides on human tuberculosis strain with multiple drug resistance. Journal of Microbial and Biochemical Technology. 2017;**9**:293-300. DOI: 10.4172/1948-5948.1000381

[27] Leonova NV. Study of the combined effect of antibacterial/antiviral agent FS-1 and antibiotics on *Staphylococcus aureus* in experiments in vitro. Meditsinski vestnik Erebuni. 2012;**49**:54-60

[28] Leonova NV. Combined action medical substance FS-1 and board spectrum antibiotic against *Staphylococcus aureus*. Veterinária. 2012;**1**:57-59

[29] Kulmanov ME, Ivanova LN, Sokolova NN, Korotetskiy IS, Kerimzhanova BF, Ilin AI. Antiflu action of the drug FS-1 in experiment with chickens. News of the National Academy of Sciences of the Republic of Kazakhstan. Series of Biological and Medical. 2015;**5**:27-35

[30] Ilin AI, Kulmanov ME, Korotetskiy IS, Islamov RA, Akhmetova GK, Lankina MV, et al. Genomic insight into mechanisms of reversion of antibiotic resistance in multidrug

resistant *Mycobacterium tuberculosis* induced by a nanomolecular iodine-containing complex FS-1. Frontiers in Cellular and Infection Microbiology. 2017;**7**:151. DOI: 10.3389/fcimb.2017.00151

[31] Volodina GV, Davtyan TK, Kulmanov ME, Dzhumagazieva AB, Tursunova SK, Abekova AO, et al. The effect of antibiotic-resistant and sensitive *Escherichia coli* on the production of pro-inflammatory cytokine response by human peripheral blood mononuclear cells. Journal of Clinical and Cellular Immunology. 2017;**8**:522. DOI: 10.4172/2155-9899.1000522

[32] Yuldasheva G, Argirova R, Ilin A. Inhibition of HIV-1 integrase active catalytic center by molecular iodine complexes with bioorganic ligands and lithium halogenides. Journal of AIDS and Clinical Research. 2015;**6**:2-6. DOI: 10.1007/978-1-4899-7699-4_10

[33] Kulmanov ME, Kerimzhanova BF, Chernousova LN, Bocharova IV, Lepekha LN, Ilin AI. Efficiency of the new medication of FS-1 in the treatment of experimental tuberculosis. Tuberculosis and Lung Diseases. 2015;**12**:50-56

[34] Kalykova AS, Vetchy D, Sakipova ZB. Development of tablet medical form containing substance FS-1. Research Journal of Pharmaceutical, Biological and Chemical Sciences. 2015;**6**:1610-1615

[35] Ilin A, Kerimzhanova B, Leonova NV, Grushina T, Meka-Mechenko T. Antibacterial activity spectrum of FS-1 medical agent. In: Proceedings of the International Conference Discovery and Development of New Anti-Infection Drugs. 17-19 September 2014. Almaty: SCAID; 2014. pp. 108-110

[36] Ilin AI, Kulmanov ME, Korotetskiy IS, Akhmetova GK, Lankina MV, Shvidko SV, et al. Complete genome sequence of multidrug-resistant clinical isolate *Mycobacterium tuberculosis* 187.0, used to study the effect of drug susceptibility reversion by the new medicinal drug FS-1. Genome Announcements. 2015;**3**:e01272-e01215. DOI: 10.1128/genomeA.01272-15

[37] Kassymbekova S, Kerimzhanova B, Ilyin A. Influences of FS-1 medicine on the cytoplasmatic membrane of *E. coli*. News of the National Academy of Sciences of the Republic of Kazakhstan Series of Biological and Medical. 2016;**2**:28-33

[38] Ordway DJ, Shanley CA, Caraway ML, Orme EA, Bucy DS, Hascall-Dove L, et al. Evaluation of standard chemotherapy in the guinea pig model of tuberculosis. Antimicrobial Agents and Chemotherapy. 2010;**54**:1820-1833. DOI: 10.1128/AAC.01521-09

[39] Tam A, Shemesh M, Wormser U, Sintov A, Steinberg D. Effect of different iodine formulations on the expression and activity of *Streptococcus mutans* glucosyltransferase and fructosyltransferase in biofilm and planktonic environments. The Journal of Antimicrobial Chemotherapy. 2006;**57**:865-871. DOI: 10.1093/jac/dkl085

[40] Oduwole KO, Glynn AA, Molony DC, Murray D, Rowe S, Holland LM, et al. Anti-biofilm activity of sub-inhibitory povidone-iodine concentrations against *Staphylococcus*

epidermidis and *Staphylococcus aureus*. Journal of Orthopaedic Research. 2010;**28**:1252-1256. DOI: 10.1002/jor.21110

[41] Korotetskiy IS, Shilov SV, Shvidko SV, Jumagaziyeva AB, Suldina NA, Korotetskaya NV, et al. Transcriptional response of the multidrug resistant *Staphylococcus aureus* following FS-1 exposure. Eurasian Journal of Applied Biotechnology. 2017;**3**:43-48

[42] Gluck U, Martin U, Bosse B, Reimer K, Mueller S. A clinical study on the tolerability of a liposomal povidone-iodine nasal spray: Implications for further development. Journal for Otorhinolaryngology and Its Related Specialties. 2007;**69**:92-99. DOI: 10.1159/000097758

[43] Ilin A, Kulmanov M, Nersesyan A, Stopper H. Genotoxic activity of the new pharmaceutical FS-1 in Salmonella/microsome test and mouse lymphoma L5178Y cells. Journal of BUON. 2015;**20**:595-601

[44] Kalykova A, Kustova T, Sakipova Z, Ibragimova N, Islamov R, Vetchý D, et al. Acute and subchronic toxicity studies of the original drug FS-1. Acta Veterinaria. 2016;**85**:009-016. DOI: 10.2754/avb201685010009

[45] Nersesyan A, Ilin A, Kulmanov M, Muradyan R, Parsadanyan G, Zalinyan G, et al. Investigations of genotoxic activity of the antimicrobial/antiviral agent FS-1 in rodents by means of the micronucleus and the comet assays. Archive of Oncology. 2011;**19**:55-58. DOI: 10.2298/AOO1104055N

[46] Ilin A, Ivanova L, Kerimzhanova B, Sokolova N. Cytotoxicity nanostructured ionics complexes in vitro. In: Proceedings of XLVIII International Scientific-Practical Conference "Scholarly Discussion: Innovations of the Modern World". 15 April 2014; Moscow: Internauka; 2014. pp. 97-105

[47] Islamov RA, Kustova TS, Ilin AI. Preclinical toxicity of new pharmaceutical substance FS-1. In: Proceedings of the International Conference Discovery and Development of New Anti-Infection Drugs. 17-19 September 2014. Almaty: SCAID; 2014. p. 172

[48] Islamov RA, Paretcskay NA, Kustova TS. Toxicokinetics of a new pharmaceutical substance FS-1 in rats. In: Proceedings of the International Conference Discovery and Development of New Anti-Infection Drugs. 17-19 September 2014. Almaty: SCAID; 2014. pp. 170-171

[49] Glick PL, Guglielmo BJ, Tranbaugh RF, Turley K. Iodine toxicity in a patient treated by continuous povidone-iodine mediastinal irrigation. The Annals of Thoracic Surgery. 1985;**39**:478-480. DOI: 10.1016/S0003-4975(10)61965-0

[50] Sherer TT, Thrall KD, Bull RJ. Comparison of toxicity induced by iodine and iodide in male and female rats. Journal of Toxicology and Environmental Health. 1991;**32**:89-101. DOI: 10.1080/15287399109531467

[51] National Research Council. Mineral Tolerance of Animals. 2nd ed. Washington, DC: The National Academies Press; 2005. 496 p. DOI: 10.17226/11309

[52] Yang XF, Xu J, Hou XH, Guo HL, Hao LP, Yao P, et al. Developmental toxic effects of chronic exposure to high doses of iodine in the mouse. Reproductive Toxicology. 2006;**22**:725-730. DOI: 10.1016/j.reprotox.2006.05.010

[53] Smith SM, Flentke GR, Garic A. Avian models in teratology and developmental toxicology. Methods in Molecular Biology (Clifton, NJ). 2012;**889**:85-103. DOI: 10.1007/978-1-61779-867-2_7

[54] Ivanova L. Antiviral activity of the medical substance FS-1 experiments in ovo. Izvestiya Natsionalьnoy Akademii Nauk Kyirgyizskoy Respubliki. 2015;**4**:34-41

[55] Chandra AK, Chakraborty A. Influence of iodine in excess on seminiferous tubular structure and epididymal sperm character in male rats. Environmental Toxicology. 2017;**32**:1823-1835. DOI: 10.1002/tox.22405

[56] Dimasi JA. Risks in new drug development: approval success rates for investigational drugs. Clinical Pharmacology and Therapeutics. 2001;**69**:297-307

[57] Adkinson NFJ, Essayan D, Gruchalla R, Haggerty H, Kawabata T, Sandler JD, et al. Task force report: Future research needs for the prevention and management of immune-mediated drug hypersensitivity reactions. The Journal of Allergy and Clinical Immunology. 2002;**109**:461-478. DOI: 10.1067/mai.2002.122214

[58] Ohtani T, Mizuashi M, Ito Y, Aiba S. Cadexomer as well as cadexomer iodine induces the production of proinflammatory cytokines and vascular endothelial growth factor by human macrophages. Experimental Dermatology. 2007;**16**:318-323. DOI: 10.1111/j.1600-0625.2006.00532.x

[59] Kulmanov ME, Bogdanov AY, Bogdanova TM, Dubeshko SY, Kalyikova AS, et al. The study of allergic activity of pharmaceutical drug of FS-1. Gigiena, epidemiologiya i immunologiya. 2009;**3**:86-92

[60] Kulmanov ME, Bogdanov AY, Bogdanova TM, Kalyikova AS, Dubeshko SY, et al. The study of immunotoxicity of pharmaceutical drug of FS-1. Zdorove i bolezn. 2009;**4**:138-149

[61] Kalykova AS, Barinov DV, Sakipova ZB, Vetchy D. Use of the direct compression method in the development of FS-1 tablets technology. Vestnik KazNMU. 2013;**5**:111-112

[62] Barinov DV, Kalykova AS, Sakipova ZB. Identification of FS-1 substance by spectral methods. Vestnik Karagandinskogo niversiteta, seriya Himiya. 2015;**1**:26-30

[63] USDHH (United States Department of Health and Human Services). Toxicological profile for iodine. Agency for Toxic Substances and Disease Registry. 2004. Available from: http://www.atsdr.cdc.gov/toxprofiles/tp158.pdf. [Accessed: June 10, 2018]

[64] Markou K, Georgopoulos N, Kyriazopoulou V, Vagenakis AG. Iodine-induced hypothyroidism. Thyroid. 2001;**11**:501-510. DOI: 10.1089/105072501300176462

[65] Wolff J, Chaikoff IL. The inhibitory action of excessive iodide upon the synthesis of diiodotyrosine and of thyroxine in the thyroid gland of the normal rat. Endocrinology. 1948;**43**:174-179. DOI: 10.1210/endo-43-3-174

[66] Eng PH, Cardona GR, Fang SL, Previti M, Alex S, Carrasco N, et al. Escape from the acute Wolff-Chaikoff effect is associated with a decrease in thyroid sodium/iodide symporter messenger ribonucleic acid and protein. Endocrinology. 1999;**140**:3404-3410. DOI: 10.1210/endo.140.8.6893

[67] Larsen PR, Davies TF, Schlumberger MJ, Hay ID. Thyroid physiology and diagnostic evaluation of patients with thyroid disorders. In: Larsen PR, Kronenberg HM, Melmed S, Polonsky KS, editors. Williams Textbook of Endocrinology. 10th ed. Philadelphia: WB Saunders Company. pp. 331-373

Chapter 8

Clinical Relevance of Medicinal Plants and Foods of Vegetal Origin on the Activity of Cytochrome P450

Xóchitl S. Ramírez-Gómez,
Sandra N. Jiménez-García, Vicente Beltrán Campos,
Esmeralda Rodríguez Miranda,
Gabriel Herrera Pérez and Rafael Vargas-Bernal

Additional information is available at the end of the chapter

http://dx.doi.org/10.5772/intechopen.79971

Abstract

Drug metabolism is a pharmacokinetic process whose main objective is to modify the chemical structure of drugs to easily excretable compounds. This process is carried out through phase I and phase II reactions. The enzymes of cytochrome P450 (CYP450) participate in phase I reactions, and their activity can be inhibited or induced by xenobiotics. The aim of this chapter is to study the clinical relevance of the induction and inhibition of CYP450, by describing the effect that some bioactive compounds present in medicinal plants or foods can modify, either increasing or decreasing the activity of CYP450 enzymes and with it modify the bioavailability and depuration of drugs. Examples will be described on the interaction of medicinal plants and foods of vegetal origin that when combined with some drugs can generate toxicity or therapeutic failure; this will allow gathering relevant information on the adequate pharmacological management in different clinical situations.

Keywords: cytochrome P450, drug metabolism, medicinal plants, foods of vegetal origin toxicity, therapeutic failure

1. Introduction

When a patient is in pharmacological treatment, and at some point a pharmacological response different from the expected one is observed, it is possible to think that a pharmacological interaction occurred. This occurs when a drug is administered or consumed in combination with other drugs, foods, or medicinal plants. In this context, changes in responses to drugs can be positive or negative for the patient. However, it is of particular interest to study the negative changes in pharmacological responses such as intoxication or therapeutic failure.

In this chapter, we focus on describing the effect of the interaction between drugs, medicinal plants, and foods of vegetable origin on the activity of cytochrome P450. Due to the natural products may modify the plasmatic concentrations of the drugs, either by inhibition or induction enzymatic, respectively.

In clinical practice, it is very important to know this topic to identify which medicinal plants and foods of vegetable origin should not be consumed when the patient is in pharmacological treatment and to avoid suffering a change in the response to medications that they consume by prescription and that could put their lives at risk.

2. General aspect of pharmacokinetics

To understand the effect of the chemical compounds, present in some medicinal plants and foods of vegetable origin on the activity of cytochrome P450 (CYP450), we will start with a brief description of the pharmacokinetics because the CYP450 participates in the phase I reactions of drug metabolism.

Pharmacokinetics is the branch of pharmacology that is responsible for studying and explaining the processes by which drugs are absorbed, distributed, metabolized, and eliminated from organism [1, 2]. It is important to know these pharmacokinetics processes and how they influence the bioavailability of drugs [2].

Bioavailability refers to the amount of drug found in the bloodstream and is available to exert its pharmacological effect [3]. However, if the plasma quantity of a drug is modified, the pharmacological response will be modified [1–3]. The four pharmacokinetic processes influence the bioavailability of the drugs. In the process of metabolism, the plasma concentrations of the drugs can be modified, either by inhibition or by induction of different CYP isoenzymes, as shown in **Figure 1**.

The following example makes it easier to understand the importance of adherence to treatment to avoid fluctuations in plasmatic concentration. When patients are in pharmacological treatment, it is important that dosage regimen be complied. For example, if the prescription is 500 mg of acetaminophen every 8 h, this patient should be taken exactly three tablets of 500 mg of acetaminophen per day.

In order for patient has an adequate pharmacological response to acetaminophen, and a lower probability of presenting adverse effects or therapeutic failure, the amount of drug and the time of administration indicated in each shot must be respected. If, patient modifies any of these two variables, the plasma concentration of the drug changes and with it its response also changes [4].

When a single dose of drug is administered orally, after a certain time, the plasma concentrations of the drug are enlarged until reaching a maximum level. This maximum point is known as maximum plasma concentration (C_{max}), and it is reached in a determined maximum

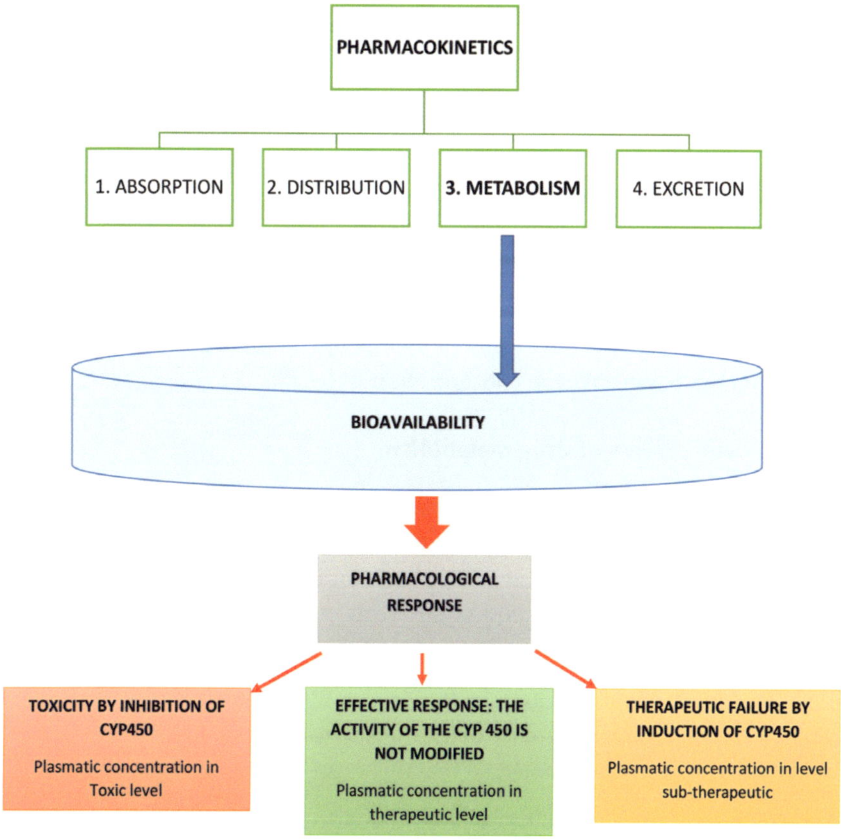

Figure 1. Effect of drug metabolism on the pharmacological response.

time (t_{max}). These parameters are specific for each drug [6]. The C_{max} of a drug is within the therapeutic range [4].

On the other hand, after several administrations of a drug, the final concentration begins to increase due to the remainder of the previous dose, until reaching a constant concentration called the equilibrium state [1]. Steady state is usually achieved after four to five half-lives [1, 2]. The half-life ($t_{1/2}$) is defined as the time required by a drug to decrease its initial concentration by half [1].

In the equilibrium state, the drug plasmatic concentrations are within the range of therapeutic effect. If the patient suspends the administration of the drug, the plasma levels fall to concentrations below the therapeutic level causing therapeutic failure. Generally, the elimination of a drug is carried out after four to five half-lives [1–3].

When the patient does not remember if took the dose of the drug and decides to take the dose thinks was needed, the concentration of that drug will accumulate, then the plasma concentration reaches levels above the therapeutic concentration, and additionally, some signs of toxicity begin to appear [5].

In this chapter, we will focus on describing the effect that some compounds present in medicinal plants and some foods of vegetable origin can have on the activity of cytochrome P450 enzymes. The World Health Organization (WHO) estimates that more than 80% of the population of developed and underdeveloped countries use medicinal plants as a first resource for their health care and, on the other hand, there is a context cultural acceptance of the traditional practice with herbs, which makes its use popular and that in many cases patients combine their pharmacological treatment with herbal treatment [6–10].

On the other hand, the consumption of certain foods of vegetable origin with nutraceutical properties has increased considerably in recent years, especially to treat and prevent conditions such as cancer, diabetes, hypertension, hypercholesterolemia, obesity, among others. Therefore, by combining these foods with the pharmacological treatment indicated in the abovementioned conditions, they can significantly modify the plasma levels of some drugs and put the patient's life at risk, either due to therapeutic failure (decrease in plasma concentration) or toxicity (increased plasma concentration) [11–15].

2.1. Pharmacokinetic process of drug metabolism

The drugs are defined chemically as acids or weak bases, and during the absorption process, the nonionized fraction of a drug is the one that crosses the biological membranes, due to its lipid solubility. Until the condition of lipid solubility is not lost, the drug will continue remaining in the body, by means of processes of reabsorption at the renal level or the enterohepatic circuit and redistribution from drug deposits in adipose tissue [16–19].

If this lipid solubility condition is not lost, the drug will not be able to be eliminated [2, 18]. Fortunately, the pharmacokinetic process of the metabolism helps to modify the chemical structure of drugs into structures more polar, so that these can be more easily excreted [2, 18, 19].

The main organ that participates in the metabolism of drugs and other xenobiotics is the liver. However, other tissues also have metabolic capacity such as the gastrointestinal tract, lungs, skin, kidneys, and brain [20–23].

The functional unit of this organ is the hepatocyte, and it contains different enzymes that are in the mitochondria, smooth and rough reticulum membrane, cytosol, etc. [23].

During this process of drug metabolism, the following may occur:

1. Transform to a more active molecule [1–3].
2. Transform to give biological activity (prodrug) [1–3].
3. Transform to an inactive molecule [1–3].
4. Transform to a toxic molecule [1–3].

It is important to mention that there are drugs that do not transform. Their chemical structure is not modified, and they are eliminated unaltered [2].

2.1.1. *Effect of metabolism of the first step*

When drugs are administered orally, they suffer a phenomenon of elimination prior to the process *per se* of the metabolism. This effect is known as first-pass metabolism and occurs in the epithelial cells of the gastrointestinal tract mainly in the small intestine [24]. Subsequently, the amount of drug that was not biotransformed enters the liver through the portal circulation, and there in the hepatocytes the metabolism process *per se* is carried out [24]. The amount of drug remaining after liver extraction is bioavailable to give an adequate pharmacological response. It is important not to modify this bioavailability because the effective doses of the drugs used in the clinical ready are considered as the effect of metabolism of the first step. Above all, caution should be exercised in drugs with a narrow safety margin, such as barbiturates [1, 2].

2.1.2. Enterohepatic circuit

When drugs are biotransformed by phase I reactions, and the molecule obtained is not polar enough to be eliminated, their biotransformation continues through phase II reactions. In this phase, the metabolites are generally conjugated with glucuronide acid, giving a polar molecule with a higher molecular weight [1, 2]. These conjugates are secreted from the hepatocyte into the bile and stored there in the form of a drug-glucuronide complex; when the bile is secreted in the intestine by some stimulus, the drug-bile complex is eliminated through the feces [25]. However, intestinal microorganisms produce various enzymes, such as beta-glucuronidases, which break the bond between the drug and glucuronide acid, leaving the drug free again, where it can be reabsorbed through the small intestine and enter the general circulation. In this case, the half-life of the drugs is increased [25].

2.1.3. Factors that affect the metabolism of drugs

2.1.3.1. Physiological factors: age and pregnancy

In children and older adults, the metabolic rate is decreased compared to the metabolic rate of a young adult [1]. In the child, the microsomal enzymes are not yet fully induced [26]. In elderly people, the number of hepatocytes and blood flow that reaches this organ is reduced [27]. So, there are fewer cytochrome P450 enzymes available to metabolize drugs. In pregnancy, there is greater hepatic flow and greater activity of cytochrome P450, which increases the metabolic rate [28].

2.1.3.2. Pathological factors: liver disease

The number of hepatocytes decreases, and the metabolic rate also decreases. In addition, there is an increase in the plasmatic concentrations and half-life of drugs. Therefore, it is necessary to adjust the dose, to prevent toxicity [2].

2.1.3.3. Drugs, medicinal plants, and foods

Some drugs and phytochemical compounds present in medicinal plants and foods of plant origin can induce or inhibit the activity of cytochrome P450 [29].

2.2. Phases of drug metabolism

Biotransformation reactions of drugs are divided into reactions of phase I or functionalization and reactions of phase II or conjugation [2].

The chemical reactions of phase I allow the introduction of functional groups such as –OH, –COOH, –SH, –O–, or $-NH_2$. Phase I reactions are very simple chemical reactions such as oxidation, reduction, hydrolysis, alkylation, and dealkylation [2]. Of these chemical reactions, the most important in the metabolism of drugs and that occur more frequently are the oxidation reactions performed by the cytochrome P450 enzymes (CYP450). These enzymes are located mainly in the smooth endoplasmic reticulum [1, 2].

When the addition of the functional groups (–OH, –COOH, –SH, –O–, $-NH_2$) to the drug molecule is not enough to transform it to a more polar molecule, the molecule continues its modification through reactions of phase II. Phase II reactions are called also conjugation reactions. In these reactions, the molecule of the drug or metabolite previously formed in the reactions of phase I is conjugated with a large molecule of polar nature (hydrophilic) as the acid glucuronide, or acetyl Co-A, glycine, glutathione, phosphoadenosyl phosphosulfate, and S-adenosylmethionine [2]. These reactions are carried out by means of specific enzymes called transferases that are generally located in the microsomes and in the cytosol [1–3].

2.3. Role of cytochrome P450 (CYP450) in drug metabolism

Cytochrome P450 (CYP450) is a superfamily of enzymes that contain a heme group, so they are hemoproteins. The iron in the heme group is reduced and forms complexes with the carbon monoxide that absorbs light at a wavelength of 450 nm [30]. They have identified more than 8700 genes that code for their proteins and are found in eukaryotic and prokaryotic cells [31]. They are responsible for metabolizing or biotransforming endogenous substances in the body such as hormones, and different xenobiotics such as drugs. These enzymes perform oxidation reactions and participate in the phase I reactions of drug metabolism [1–3]. They are also known as mixed function oxidases or monooxygenases; they require a reducing agent such as NADPH and molecular oxygen [32].

They have different patterns of specificity for the substrate; for example, acetaminophen is a substrate of both CYP1A2 and CYP2E1, while halogenated anesthetics are substrate only of CYP2E1 [2, 34–36]. This enzyme system is found in different tissues such as kidney, lung, skin, brain, adrenal cortex, placenta, testicles, and other tissues, but the liver and small intestine are the organs that have more CYP450 [33, 34].

2.3.1. Nomenclature of CYP450

The CYP450 is grouped into families and subfamilies depending on the analogy in their amino acid sequences, such that CYPs that present 40% homology in their amino acids belong to a family, and when the analogy is greater than 55%, they form a subfamily, are named with the prefix CYP, and followed by the family number, a capital letter indicating the subfamily, and a number that marks the individual form: for example, CYP1A1, in this way, represents the individual form 1 of subfamily A of family 1 [35]. Eighteen families, 42 subfamilies, and more than 50 individual genes of human origin have been described. However, the most important in the metabolism of drugs are CYP1A1/2, CYP1B1, CYP2A6, CYP2B6, CYP2C9,

CYP2D6, CYP2E1, CYP3A4,5,7 [1–3]. CYP3A4,5,7 is the most abundant and participates in the metabolism of more than 50% of the drugs currently used in the clinic [1–3, 35].

2.4. Induction and Enzymatic inhibition

Many substances such as drugs, environmental toxins, and phytochemicals present in medicinal plants and some foods of plant origin contain substances that act as inhibitors or inducers of cytochrome P450 enzymes; this induction and inhibition can be strong or weak so it can sometimes have relevant clinical implications such as producing toxicity or therapeutic failure [36].

Enzymatic induction refers to the increase of enzymes and/or their activity. Additionally, it increases the metabolic rate of CYP450, and therefore, the concentrations of the drug in blood will decrease, which can cause a decrease in pharmacological effects and with it a therapeutic failure (**Figure 2**) [37].

In enzymatic inhibition, the number of enzymes and/or their activity decreases. There are fewer enzymes available to biotransform the drugs and increase their plasma levels with each administration of the drug will produce toxicity (**Figure 2**) [33].

It is important not to induce or inhibit the activity of CYP450; they directly influence the bioavailability of the drugs. On the other hand, the genetic polymorphism of CYP450 is also responsible for the variability in the response to drugs between each individual [34, 35]. Genetic variability, especially of CYP2C9, CYP2C19, CYP2D6, and CYP3A5, is known to have an important clinical impact on drugs that are metabolized by these enzymes [38–40].

2.5. Effect of bioactive compounds of medicinal plants and foods of vegetable origin on the activity of CYP450

In the literature, there is a lot of information about the effect of drugs to inhibit or induce certain CYP450 isoenzymes. Recently the study of the effect of some phytochemical components that are present in medicinal plants and foods of vegetable origin on the activity of CYP450 has been increasing, because the population makes use of herbal medicine in its traditional practice and, on the other hand, it consumes foods with nutraceutical properties, either to prevent or to control any disease.

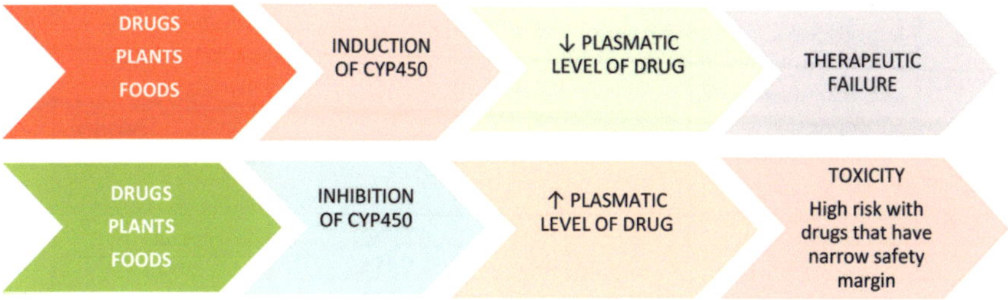

Figure 2. Effect of medicinal plants and foods of vegetable origin on CYP450 activity.

Medicinal plant	Tradicional uses	Phytochemistry compounds	Activity on CYP450	Clinical effect on substrates of CYP450	References
Artemisia annua L.	Antimalaria effect	Artemisinin	↑CYP2C19	↓Plasmatic concentration of I	[3, 41, 42]
Cimicifuga racemosa	Are used as a hormone replacement and antiinflammatory	Triterpene glycosides Fukinolic acid Cimicifugic acid A Cimicifugic acid B	↓CYP1A2 ↓CYP2D6 ↓CYP2C9 ↓CYP3A4	↑Plasmatic concentration of II ↑Plasmatic concentration of III ↑Plasmatic concentration of IV ↑Plasmatic concentration of V	[3, 43]
Centella asiatica	Used for wound healing and maintaining normal blood pressure.	Flavonoids: Quercetin Kaempferol	↓CYP2D6 ↓CYP2C9 ↓CYP3A4	↑Plasmatic concentration of III ↑Plasmatic concentration of IV ↑Plasmatic concentration of V	[3, 44, 45]
Curcuma longa	Antiinflammatory, anticancer and antiarthritic effect.	Curcuminoids: Curcumin Methoxycurcumin, Bisdemethoxy-curcumin	↓CYP1A2 ↑CYP2A6 ↓CYP2C9 ↓CYP3A4	↑Plasmatic concentration of II ↓Plasmatic concentration of VI ↑Plasmatic concentration of IV ↑Plasmatic concentration of V	[3, 46–48]
Echinacea purpurea (L.)	It is used to treat colds, upper respiratory infections, and dermatologic issues	Cichoric acid Caftaric acid Echinacoside Alkylamides	↑CYP1A2 ↓CYP3A4	↓Plasmatic concentration of II ↑Plasmatic concentration of V	[3, 49, 50]
Garcinia cambogia	Obesity treatment	Extract crude	↓CYP2B6	↑Plasmatic concentration of VII	[3, 51]
Gardenia jasminoides Ellis.	Is used as an antioxidant, hypoglycemic, antithrombotic, antiinflammatory, antidepression effect, and improved sleeping quality	Geniposide Genipin	↑CYP2D6 ↓CYP2C19 ↓CYP3A4	↓Plasmatic concentration of III ↑Plasmatic concentration of I ↑Plasmatic concentration of V	[3, 52, 53]
Gingko biloba	It is used as an anti-hypertensive as well as to treat macular degeneration and tinnitus. Are effective in treating cerebral infarction	Ginkgolide A Ginkgolide B Bilobalide Quercetin kaempferol	↓CYP2B6 ↑CYP1A2 ↑CYP3A4	↑Plasmatic concentration of VII ↓Plasmatic concentration of II ↓Plasmatic concentration of V	[3, 54–56]

Medicinal plant	Tradicional uses	Phytochemistry compounds	Activity on CYP450	Clinical effect on substrates of CYP450	References
Panax ginseng	Is believed to enhance cognitive ability and to lower blood sugar levels Ginsenosides and gintonin Ginsenoside F2 and protopanaxadiol	Ginsenosides	↓CYP2C9 ↓CYP3A4	↑Plasmatic concentration of IV ↑Plasmatic concentration of V	[3, 57]
Camellia sinensis	It is consumed to treat cancer, cardiovascular disease, dyslipidemia, inflammation, and weight loss	Catechin (-)-Epigallocatechin -3-gallate	↓CYP1A2 ↓CYP2B6 ↓CYP2C8 ↓CYP2C9 ↓CYP2D6 ↓CYP3A4	↑Plasmatic concentration of II ↑Plasmatic concentration of VII ↑Plasmatic concentration of VIII ↑Plasmatic concentration of IV ↑Plasmatic concentration of III ↑Plasmatic concentration of V	[3, 58–60]
Piper methysticum	Anxiolytic effect	Flavokawain A	↑CYP2C9 ↓CYP1A2 ↓CYP3A4	↓Plasmatic concentration of IV ↑Plasmatic concentration of II ↑Plasmatic concentration of V	[3, 61–64]
Hypericum perforatum	Is used to treat anxiety and depression	Hyperforin	↑CYP2C9 ↑CYP3A4	↓Plasmatic concentration of IV ↓Plasmatic concentration of V	[3, 65–67]

I: Omeprazole, pantoprazole, diazepam, S-mephenytoin, amitriptyline, carisoprodol, citalopram, chloramphenicol, clomipramine, cyclophosphamide, indomethacin, moclobemide, nelfinavir, propranolol, progesterone.

II: Acetaminophen, amitriptyline, phenacetin, tacrine, theophylline, tamoxifen, (R)warfarin, caffeine, verapamil, ondansetron, haloperidol, naproxen, propanolol.

III: Propoxyphene, codeine, oxycodone, dextromethorphan, clozapine, timolol, tamoxifen, tramadol, seleglinide, fluoxetine, phenformin, paroxetine, risperidone, metoprolol, tricyclic antidepressants.

IV: Amitriptyline, celcoxib, ibuprofen, diclofenac, meloxicam, hexobarbital, losartan, S-warfarin, fluvastation, phenytoin, tolbutamide, glipizide, glibenclamide, fluoxetine, tamoxifen.

V: Acetaminophen, amiodarone, cisapride, astemizole, cocaine, cyclosporine, dapsone, diazepam, dihydroergotamine, diltiacem, felodipine, nifedipine, erythromycin, indinavir, lidocaine, methadone, miconazole, quinidine, paclitaxel, mifepristone, spironolactone, verapamil, trazolam, desametaxone, ritonavir, lovastatin, hydrocortisone.

VI: Nicotine.

VII: Bupropion, cyclophosphamide, efavirenz, ifosfamide, methadone.

VIII: Paclitaxel, torsemide, amodiaquine, cerivastatin, repaglinide.

Table 1. Effect of medicinal plants on CYP450 activity.

Fruit or vegetable	Phytochemistry compound	Activity on CYP450	Clinical effect on substrates of CYP450	References
Broccoli	Sulforaphane	↑CYP1A2 ↓CYP2D6	↓Plasmatic concentration of II ↑Plasmatic concentration of III	[3, 68, 69]
Grapefruit	Furanocoumarin	↓CYP3A4	↑Plasmatic concentration of V	[3, 65, 70, 71]
Pomegranate	Flavonoids Tannins Phenolic acids	↓CYP2C9 ↓CYP3A4	↑Plasmatic concentration of IV ↑Plasmatic concentration of V	[3, 72]
Sevillian orange	Furanocoumarin	↓CYP3A4	↑Plasmatic concentration of V	[3, 73]
Star fruit	Catechin Epicatechin	↓CYP3A4	↑Plasmatic concentration of V	[3, 74–76]

II: Acetaminophen, amitriptyline, phenacetin, tacrine, theophylline, tamoxifen, (R)warfarin, caffeine, verapamil, ondansetron, haloperidol, naproxen, propanolol.

III: Propoxyphene, codeine, oxycodone, dextromethorphan, clozapine, timolol, tamoxifen, tramadol, seleglinide, fluoxetine, phenformin, paroxetine, risperidone, metoprolol, tricyclic antidepressants.

IV: Amitriptyline, celcoxib, ibuprofen, diclofenac, meloxicam, hexobarbital, losartan, S-warfarin, fluvastation, phenytoin, tolbutamide, glipizide, glibenclamide, fluoxetine, tamoxifen.

V: Acetaminophen, amiodarone, cisapride, astemizole, cocaine, cyclosporine, dapsone, diazepam, dihydroergotamine, diltiacem, felodipine, nifedipine, erythromycin, indinavir, lidocaine, methadone, miconazole, quinidine, paclitaxel, mifepristone, spironolactone, verapamil, trazolam, desametaxone, ritonavir, lovastatin, hydrocortisone.

Table 2. Effect of fruits or vegetables on CYP450 activity.

Tables 1 and **2** show the effect of the phytochemical compounds present in medicinal plants and foods of vegetable origin. We mentioned principally those natural products that have an important effect on the induction and inhibition of different CYP450 isoenzymes and that have clinical relevance to produce toxicity or therapeutic failure.

3. Conclusions

The induction and inhibition of CYP450, by some bioactive compounds present in medicinal plants or foods, can modify the bioavailability of drugs. The changes in the bioavailability are important in the efficacy and safety of pharmacological management. It is important to consider that when a patient will be in a pharmacologic treatment, the patient should not use any medicinal plants or foods of vegetable origin that can induce or inhibit any CYP450 isoenzymes.

Especially, they should not use the St. John's wort and grapefruit, as their phytochemical compounds have a potent effect to induce or inhibit, respectively, the activity of CYP3A4 with important clinical relevance.

Author details

Xóchitl S. Ramírez-Gómez[1]*, Sandra N. Jiménez-García[2], Vicente Beltrán Campos[1], Esmeralda Rodríguez Miranda[3], Gabriel Herrera Pérez[4] and Rafael Vargas-Bernal[4]

*Address all correspondence to: xosofira2002@yahoo.com.mx

1 Department of Clinical Nursing, Division of Health Sciences and Engineering, University of Guanajuato, Celaya, Guanajuato, Mexico

2 Department of Nursing and Obstetrics, Division of Health Sciences and Engineering, University of Guanajuato, Celaya, Guanajuato, Mexico

3 Department of Medicine and Nutrition, Division of Health Sciences, University of Guanajuato, León, Guanajuato, Mexico

4 Department of Materials Engineering, Instituto Tecnológico Superior de Irapuato, Irapuato, Guanajuato, Mexico

References

[1] Brunton LL, Chabner BA, Knollman B. Goodman & Gilman's The Pharmacological Basis of Therapeutics. 12th ed. United States: McGraw-Hill; 2012. pp. 123-143

[2] Katzung BG, Masters SB, Trevor AJ. Basic & Clinical Pharmacology. 12th ed. United States: McGraw-Hill; 2013. pp. 37-68

[3] Flórez J, Armijo JA, Mediavilla A. Human Pharmacology. 6th ed. Barcelona, Spain: McGraw-Hill; 2014. pp. 46-105

[4] Mehrotra N, Gupta M, Kovar A, Meibohm B. The role of pharmacokinetics and pharmacodynamics in phosphodiesterase-5 inhibitor therapy. International Journal of Impotence Research. 2007;**19**:253-264. DOI: 10.1038/sj.ijir.3901522

[5] Chawla PK, Udwadia ZF, Soman R, Mahashur AA, Amale RA, Dherai AJ, Lokhande RV, Naik PR, Ashavaid TF. Importance of therapeutic drug monitoring of rifampicin. The Journal of the Association of Physicians of India. 2016;**64**:68-72

[6] World Health Organization. Traditional Medicine Strategy 2014-2023 [Internet]. Available from: http://apps.who.int/medicinedocs/documents/s21201en/s21201en.pdf [Accessed: April 01, 2018]

[7] Brewer CT, Chen T. Hepatotoxicity of herbal supplements mediated by modulation of cytochrome P450. International Journal of Molecular Sciences. 2017;**18**:E2353. DOI: 10.3390/ijms18112353

[8] Hua S, Zhang Y, Liu J, Dong L, Huang J, Lin D, Fu X. Ethnomedicine, phytochemistry and pharmacology of *Smilax glabra*: An important traditional Chinese medicine. The American Journal of Chinese Medicine. 2018;**46**:261-297. DOI: 10.1142/S0192415X18500143

[9] Cruz EC, Andrade-Cetto A. Ethnopharmacological field study of the plants used to treat type 2 diabetes among the Cakchiquels in Guatemala. Journal of Ethnopharmacology. 2005;**159**:238-244. DOI: 10.1016/j.jep.2014.11.021

[10] Martínez-Francés V, Hahn E, Ríos S, Rivera D, Reich E, Vila R, Cañiqueral S. Ethnopharmacological and chemical characterization of *Salvia* species used in Valencian traditional herbal preparations. Frontiers in Pharmacology. 2017;**8**:467. DOI: 10.3389/fphar.2017.00467

[11] Alfano A, Corsuto L, Finamore R, Savarese M, Ferrara F, Falco S, Santabarbara G, De Rosa M, Schiraldi C. Valorization of olive mill wastewater by membrane processes to recover natural antioxidant compounds for cosmeceutical and nutraceutical applications or functional foods. Antioxidants (Basel). 2018;**7**:E72. DOI: 10.3390/antiox7060072

[12] Benatrehina PA, Pan L, Naman CB, Li J, Kinghorn AD. Usage, biological activity, and safety of selected botanical dietary supplements consumed in the United States. Journal of Traditional and Complementary Medicine. 2018;**8**:267-277. DOI: 10.1016/j.jtcme.2018.01.006

[13] Maroyi A. Nutraceutical and ethnopharmacological properties of *Vangueria infausta* subsp. *infausta*. Molecules. 2018;**23**:E1089. DOI: 10.3390/molecules23051089

[14] Singh BN. Effects of food on clinical pharmacokinetics. Clinical Pharmacokinetics. 1999;**37**:213-255. DOI: 10.2165/00003088-199937030-00003

[15] Péter S, Navis G, de Borst MH, von Schacky C, van Orten-Luiten ACB, Zhernakova A, Witkamp RF, Janse A, Weber P, Bakker SJL, Eggersdorfer M. Public health relevance of drug-nutrition interactions. European Journal of Nutrition. 2017;**56**:23-36. DOI: 10.1007/s00394-017-1510-3

[16] Li ZQ, Tian S, Gu H, Wu ZG, Nyagblordzro M, Feng G, He X. In vitro-in vivo predictive dissolution-permeation-absorption dynamics of highly permeable drug extended-release tablets via drug dissolution/absorption simulating system and pH alteration. AAPS PharmSciTech. 2018;**19**:1882-1893. DOI: 10.1208/s12249-018-0996-1

[17] Romand S, Schappler J, Veuthey JL, Carrupt PA, Martel S. cIEF for rapid pKa determination of small molecules: A proof of concept. European Journal of Pharmaceutical Sciences. 2014;**63**:14-21. DOI: 10.1016/j.ejps.2014.06.016

[18] Li M, Zhang H, Chen B, Wu Y, Guan L. Prediction of pKa values for neutral and basic drugs based on hybrid artificial intelligence methods. Scientific Reports. 2018;**8**:3991. DOI: 10.1038/s41598-018-22332-7

[19] Manallack DT, Prankerd RJ, Yuriev E, Oprea TI, Chalmers DK. The significance of acid/base properties in drug discovery. Chemical Society Reviews. 2013;**42**:485-496. DOI: 10.1039/c2cs35348b

[20] Krishna DR, Klotz U. Extrahepatic metabolism of drugs in humans. Clinical Pharmacokinetics. 1994;**26**:144-160. DOI: 10.2165/00003088-199426020-00007

[21] Paine MF, Hart HL, Ludington SS, Haining RL, Rettie AE, Zeldin DC. The human intestinal cytochrome P450 "pie". Drug Metabolism and Disposition. 2006;**34**:880-886. DOI: 10.1124/dmd.105.008672

[22] Kvist AJ, Kanebratt KP, Walentinsson A, Palmgren H, O'Hara M, Björkbom A, Andersson LC, Ahlqvist M, Andersson TB. Critical differences in drug metabolic properties of human hepatic cellular models, including primary human hepatocytes, stem cell derived hepatocytes, and hepatoma cell lines. Biochemical Pharmacology. 2018;**55**:124-140. DOI: 10.1016/j.bcp.2018.06.026

[23] Sevior DK, Pelkonen O, Ahokas JT. Hepatocytes: The powerhouse of biotransformation. The International Journal of Biochemistry & Cell Biology. 2012;**44**:257-261. DOI: 10.1016/j.biocel.2011.11.011

[24] Alqahtani S, Bukhari I, Albassam A, Alenazi M. An update on the potential role of intestinal first-pass metabolism for the prediction of drug–drug interactions: The role of PBPK modeling. Expert Opinion on Drug Metabolism & Toxicology. 2018;**14**:625-634. DOI: 10.1080/17425255.2018.1482277

[25] Malik MY, Jaiswal S, Sharma A, Shukla M, Lal J. Role of enterohepatic recirculation in drug disposition: Cooperation and complications. Drug Metabolism Reviews. 2016; **48**:281-327. DOI: 10.3109/03602532.2016.1157600

[26] Stockmann C, Constance JE, Roberts JK, Olson J, Doby EH, Ampofo K, Stiers J, Spigarelli MG, Sherwin CM. Pharmacokinetics and pharmacodynamics of antifungals in children and their clinical implications. Clinical Pharmacokinetics. 2014;**53**:429-454. DOI: 10.1007/s40262-014-0139-0

[27] Turnheim K. When drug therapy gets old: Pharmacokinetics and pharmacodynamics in the elderly. Experimental Gerontology. 2003;**38**:843-853

[28] Koren G, Pariente G. Pregnancy—Associated changes in pharmacokinetics and their clinical implications. Pharmaceutical Research. 2018;**35**:61. DIO: 10.1007/s11095-018-2352-2

[29] Brewer L, Williams D. Clinically relevant drug–drug and drug–food interactions. Pharmaceutical Medicine. 2013;**27**(1):9-23. DOI: 10.1007/s40290-013-0008-4

[30] Klingenberg M. Pigments of rat liver microsomes. Archives of Biochemistry and Biophysics. 1958;**75**(2):376-386. DOI: 10.1016/0003-9861(58)90436-3

[31] Ioannides C, Lewis DF. Cytochromes P450 in the bioactivation of chemicals. Current Topics in Medicinal Chemistry. 2004;**4**:1767-1788

[32] Brewer CT, Chen T. PXR variants: The impact on drug metabolism and therapeutic responses. Acta Pharmaceutica Sinica B. 2016;**6**:441-449. DOI: 10.1016/j.apsb.2016.07.002

[33] Eagling VA, Back DJ, Barry MG. Differential inhibition of cytochrome P450 isoforms by the protease inhibitors, ritonavir, saquinavir and indinavir. British Journal of Clinical Pharmacology. 1997;**44**(2):190-194

[34] Restrepo JG, Garcia-Martín E, Martínez C, Agúndez JA. Polymorphic drug metabolism in anaesthesia. Current Drug Metabolism. 2009;**10**:236-246. DOI: 10.2174/138920009787846305

[35] Nelson DR. Cytochrome P450 nomenclature, 2004. Methods in Molecular Biology. 2006; **320**:1-10. DOI: 10.1385/1-59259-998-2:1

[36] Ding X, Kaminsky LS. Human extrahepatic cytochromes P450: Function in xenobiotic metabolism and tissue-selective chemical toxicity in the respiratory and gastrointestinal tracts. Annual Review of Pharmacology and Toxicology. 2003;**43**:149-173. DOI: 10.1146/annurev.pharmtox.43.100901.140251

[37] Tompkins LM, Wallace AD. Mechanisms of cytochrome P450 induction. Journal of Biochemical and Molecular Toxicology. 2007;**21**:176-181

[38] Zanger UM, Schwab M. Cytochrome P450 enzymes in drug metabolism: Regulation of gene expression, enzyme activities, and impact of genetic variation. Pharmacology & Therapeutics. 2013;**138**:103-141. DOI: 10.1016/j.pharmthera.2012.12.007

[39] Fanni D, Ambul R, Gerosa C, Nemolato S, Castagnola M, Van Eyken P, Faa G, Fanos V. Cytochrome P450 genetic polymorphism in neonatal drug metabolism: Role and practical consequences towards a new drug culture in neonatology. International Journal of Immunopathology and Pharmacology. 2014;**27**:5-13. DOI: 10.1177/039463201402700102

[40] Sychev DA, Ashraf GM, Svistunov AA, Maksimov ML, Tarasov VV, Chubarev VN, Otdelenov VA, Denisenko NP, Barreto GE, Aliev G. The cytochrome P450 isoenzyme and some new opportunities for the prediction of negative drug interaction in vivo. Drug Design, Development and Therapy. 2018;**12**:1147-1156. DOI: 10.2147/DDDT.S149069

[41] Misra A, Chanotiya CS, Gupta MM, Dwivedi UN, Shasany AK. Characterization of cytochrome P450 monooxygenases isolated from trichome enriched fraction of *Artemisia annua* L. leaf. Gene. 2012;**510**:193-201. DOI: 10.1016/j.gene.2012.09.015

[42] Shen Q, Chen YF, Wang T, Wu SY, Lu X, Zhang L, Zhang FY, Jiang WM, Wang GF, Tang KX. Overexpression of the cytochrome P450 monooxygenase (cyp71av1) and cytochrome P450 reductase (cpr) genes increased artemisinin content in *Artemisia annua* (Asteraceae). Genetics and Molecular Research. 2012;**11**:3298-3309. DOI: 10.4238/2012

[43] Huang Y, Jiang B, Nuntanakorn P, Kennelly EJ, Shord S, Lawal TO, Mahady GB. Fukinolic acid derivatives and triterpene glycosides from black cohosh inhibit CYP isozymes, but are not cytotoxic to Hep-G2 cells in vitro. Current Drug Safety. 2010;**5**:118-124

[44] Savai J, Varghese A, Pandita N, Chintamaneni M. Investigation of CYP3A4 and CYP2D6 interactions of *Withania somnifera* and *Centella asiatica* in human liver microsomes. Phytotherapy Research. 2015;**29**:785-790. DOI: 10.1002/ptr.5308

[45] Pan Y, Abd-Rashid BA, Ismail Z, Ismail R, Mak JW, Pook PC, Er HM, Ong CE. In vitro modulatory effects on three major human cytochrome P450 enzymes by multiple

active constituents and extracts of *Centella asiatica*. Journal of Ethnopharmacology. 2010;**130**:275-283. DOI: 10.1016/j.jep.2010.05.002

[46] Hsieh YW, Huang CY, Yang SY, Peng YH, Yu CP, Chao PD, Hou YC. Oral intake of curcumin markedly activated CYP 3A4: In vivo and ex-vivo studies. Scientific Reports. 2014;**4**:6587. DOI: 10.1038/srep06587

[47] Chen Y, Liu WH, Chen BL, Fan L, Han Y, Wang G, Hu DL, Tan ZR, Zhou G, Cao S, Zhou HH. Plant polyphenol curcumin signifcantly affects CYPIA2 and CYP2A6 activity in healthy, male Chinese volunteers. Annals of Pharmacotherapy. 2010;**44**:1038-1045. DOI: 10.1345/aph.1M533

[48] Wang Z, Sun W, Huang CK, Wang L, Xia MM, Cui X, Hu GX, Wang ZS. Inhibitory effects of curcumin on activity of cytochrome P450 2C9 enzyme in human and 2C11 in rat liver microsomes. Drug Development and Industrial Pharmacy. 2015;**41**:613-616. DOI: 10.3109/03639045.2014.886697

[49] Modarai M, Gertsch J, Suter A, Heinrich M, Kortenkamp A. Cytochrome P450 inhibitory action of Echinacea preparations differs widely and co-varies with alkylamide content. The Journal of Pharmacy and Pharmacology. 2007;**59**:567-573. DOI: 10.1211/jpp.59.4.0012

[50] Gorski JC, Huang SM, Pinto A, Hamman MA, Hilligoss JK, Zaheer NA, Desai M, Miller M, Hall SD. The effect of echinacea (*Echinacea purpurea* root) on cytochrome P450 activity in vivo. Clinical Pharmacology and Therapeutics. 2004;**75**:89-100. DOI: 10.1016/j.clpt.2003.09.013

[51] Yu JS, Choi MS, Park JS, Rehman SU, Nakamura K, Yoo HH. Inhibitory effects of *Garcinia cambogia* extract on CYP2B6 enzyme activity. Planta Medica. 2017;**83**:895-900. DOI: 10.1055/s-0043-104934

[52] Xiao W, Li S, Wang S, Ho CT. Chemistry and bioactivity of *Gardenia jasminoides*. Journal of Food and Drug Analysis. 2017;**25**:43-61. DOI: 10.1016/j.jfda.2016.11.005

[53] Gao LN, Zhang Y, Cui YL, Yan K. Evaluation of genipin on human cytochrome P450 isoenzymes and P-glycoprotein in vitro. Fitoterapia. 2014;**98**:130-136. DOI: 10.1016/j.fitote.2014.07.018

[54] Zhou XW, Ma Z, Geng T, Wang ZZ, Ding G, Yu-an B, Xiao W. Evaluation of in vitro inhibition and induction of cytochrome P450 activities by hydrolyzed ginkgolides. Journal of Ethnopharmacology. 2014;**158**(Pt A):132-139. DOI: 10.1016/j.jep.2014.10.023

[55] Lau AJ, Chang TK. Inhibition of human CYP2B6-catalyzed bupropion hydroxylation by *Ginkgo biloba* extract: Effect of terpene trilactones and flavonols. Drug Metabolism and Disposition. 2009;**37**:1931-1937. DOI: 10.1124/dmd.109.028118

[56] Deng Y, Bi HC, Zhao LZ, He F, Liu YQ, Yu JJ, Ou ZM, Ding L, Chen X, Huang ZY, Huang M, Zhou SF. Induction of cytochrome P450s by terpene trilactones and flavonoids of the *Ginkgo biloba* extract EGb 761 in rats. Xenobiotica. 2008;**38**:465-481. DOI: 10.1080/00498250701883233

[57] Xiao J, Chen D, Lin XX, Peng SF, Xiao MF, Huang WH, Wang YC, Peng JB, Zhang W, Ouyang DS, Chen Y. Screening of drug metabolizing enzymes for the ginsenoside compound K in vitro: An efficient anti-cancer substance originating from *Panax ginseng*. PLoS One. 2016;**11**:e0147183. DOI: 10.1371/journal.pone.0147183

[58] Misaka S, Miyazaki N, Fukushima T, Yamada S, Kimura J. Effects of green tea extract and (−)-epigallocatechin-3-gallate on pharmacokinetics of nadolol in rats. Phytomedicine. 2013;**20**:1247-1250. DOI: 10.1016/j.phymed.2013.07.003

[59] Albassam AA, Markowitz JS. An appraisal of drug-drug interactions with green tea (*Camellia sinensis*). Planta Medica. 2017;**83**:496-508. DOI: 10.1055/s-0043-100934

[60] Satoh T, Fujisawa H, Nakamura A, Takahashi N, Watanabe K. Inhibitory effects of eight green tea catechins on cytochrome P450 1A2, 2C9, 2D6, and 3A4 activities. Journal of Pharmacy & Pharmaceutical Sciences. 2016;**19**:188-197. DOI: 10.18433/J3MS5C

[61] Niu L, Ding L, Lu C, Zuo F, Yao K, Xu S, Li W, Yang D, Xu X. Flavokawain A inhibits cytochrome P450 in in vitro metabolic and inhibitory investigations. Journal of Ethnopharmacology. 2016;**191**:350-359. DOI: 10.1016/j.jep.2016.06.039

[62] Li Y, Mei H, Wu Q, Zhang S, Fang JL, Shi L, Guo L. Methysticin and 7,8-dihydromethysticin are two major kavalactones in Kava extract to induce CYP1A1. Toxicological Sciences. 2011;**124**:388-399. DOI: 10.1093/toxsci/kfr235

[63] Gurley BJ, Gardner SF, Hubbard MA, Williams DK, Gentry WB, Khan IA, Shah A. In vivo effects of goldenseal, kava kava, black cohosh, and valerian on human cytochrome P450 1A2, 2D6, 2E1, and 3A4/5 phenotypes. Clinical Pharmacology and Therapeutics. 2005;**77**:415-426. DOI: 10.1016/j.clpt.2005.01.009

[64] Mathews JM, Etheridge AS, Black SR. Inhibition of human cytochrome P450 activities by kava extract and kavalactones. Drug Metabolism and Disposition. 2002;**30**:1153-1157

[65] Nowack R. Review article: Cytochrome P450 enzyme, and transport protein mediated herb–drug interactions in renal transplant patients: Grapefruit juice, St John's wort—And beyond! Nephrology (Carlton). 2008;**13**:337-347. DOI: 10.1111/j.1440-1797.2008.00940.x

[66] Gurley BJ, Gardner SF, Hubbard MA, Williams DK, Gentry WB, Cui Y, Ang CY. Clinical assessment of effects of botanical supplementation on cytochrome P450 phenotypes in the elderly: St John's wort, garlic oil, *Panax ginseng* and *Ginkgo biloba*. Drugs & Aging. 2005;**22**:525-539

[67] Soleymani S, Bahramsoltani R, Rahimi R, Abdollahi M. Clinical risks of St John's wort (*Hypericum perforatum*) co-administration. Expert Opinion on Drug Metabolism & Toxicology. 2017;**13**:1047-1062. DOI: 10.1080/17425255.2017.1378342

[68] Hakooz N, Hamdan I. Effects of dietary broccoli on human in vivo caffeine metabolism: A pilot study on a group of Jordanian volunteers. Current Drug Metabolism. 2007;**8**:9-15. DOI: 10.2174/138920007779315080

[69] Vanduchova A, Tomankova V, Anzenbacher P, Anzenbacherova E. Influence of sulforaphane metabolites on activities of human drug-metabolizing cytochrome P450 and determination of sulforaphane in human liver cells. Journal of Medicinal Food. 2016;**19**:1141-1146

[70] Hanley MJ, Cancalon P, Widmer WW, Greenblatt DJ. The effect of grapefruit juice on drug disposition. Expert Opinion on Drug Metabolism & Toxicology. 2011;**7**:267-286. DOI: 10.1517/17425255.2011.553189

[71] Chen M, Zhou SY, Fabriaga E, Zhang PH, Zhou Q. Food-drug interactions precipitated by fruit juices other than grapefruit juice: An update review. Journal of Food and Drug Analysis. 2018;**26**:S61-S71. DOI: 10.1016/j.jfda.2018.01.009

[72] Singh B, Singh JP, Kaur A, Singh N. Phenolic compounds as beneficial phytochemicals in pomegranate (*Punica granatum* L.) peel: A review. Food Chemistry. 2018;**261**:75-86. DOI: 10.1016/j.foodchem.2018.04.039

[73] Molden E, Spigset O. Fruit and berries—Interactions with drugs. Tidsskrift for den Norske Lægeforening. 2007;**127**:3218-3220

[74] Zhang JW, Liu Y, Cheng J, Li W, Ma H, Liu HT, Sun J, Wang LM, He YQ, Wang Y, Wang ZT, Yang L. Inhibition of human liver cytochrome P450 by star fruit juice. Journal of Pharmacy & Pharmaceutical Sciences. 2007;**10**:496-503

[75] Hosoi S, Shimizu E, Arimori K, Okumura M, Hidaka M, Yamada M, Sakushima A. Analysis of CYP3A inhibitory components of star fruit (*Averrhoa carambola* L.) using liquid chromatography-mass spectrometry. Journal of Natural Medicines. 2008;**62**:345-348. DOI: 10.1007/s11418-008-0239-y

[76] Hidaka M, Fujita K, Ogikubo T, Yamasaki K, Iwakiri T, Okumura M, Kodama H, Arimori K. Potent inhibition by star fruit of human cytochrome P450 3A (CYP3A) activity. Drug Metabolism and Disposition. 2004;**32**:581-583. DOI: 10.1124/dmd.32.6.581

Section 4

Effects on Biological Systems: In Vivo Testing

Chapter 9

The Pragmatic Strategy to Detect Endocrine-Disrupting Activity of Xenobiotics in Food

Shui-Yuan Lu, Pinpin Lin, Wei-Ren Tsai and Chen-Yi Weng

Additional information is available at the end of the chapter

http://dx.doi.org/10.5772/intechopen.81030

Abstract

Endocrine-disrupting activity induced by xenobiotics might pose a possible health threat. Facing so many chemicals, there is an issue on how we detect them precisely and effectively. The whole embryo culture (WEC) test, an ex vivo exposure lasting 48 hours with rat embryos of 10.5 days old, is used to detect prenatal developmental toxicity. We extended the WEC function to detect the endocrine-disrupting activity induced by environmental chemicals. Results showed that in the development of rat embryo, basically 17ß-estradiol, triiodothyronine, triadimefon, penconazole, and propiconazole exhibited no significant effect on yolk sac circulatory system, allantois, flexion, heart caudal neural tube, hindbrain, midbrain, forebrain, otic system, optic system, olfactory system, maxillary process, forelimb, hind limb, yolk sac diameter, crown-rump length, head length, and developmental score. In the immunohistochemistry, the positive control of 17ß-estradiol showed positive effect for its receptor expressions. These three triazoles induced expressions of ERα and ERß in WEC. This result basically meets the mode of action that triazoles were designed to disrupt the synthesis of steroid hormone. Here we gave a strategy to detect possible endocrine-disrupting activity induced by xenobiotics in food. This strategy is quick to initiate the whole rat embryo culture with 10.5 days to detect the hormone receptors such as androgen, estrogen, thyroid, aromatase activity and its related receptors.

Keywords: whole embryo culture, xenobiotic, receptors, ex vivo, in vivo, endocrine-disrupting activity

1. Introduction

As we know, there are many pesticides identified as endocrine disruptors, but the degree of endocrine-disrupting activity (EDA) is different [1–5]. The different disrupting activities are involved in pesticide management. Because the potential endocrine-disrupting pesticides should be prohibited, low EDA will be accepted under the control of below maximum residue level (MRL). The development of new pesticide is based on its chemical functional groups for pests including fungicides, insecticides, herbicides, and others. Due to the objective of pest control of diseases, insects, and weeds, the side effect of pesticides will be appropriately managed in order not to pose risk to the human and environment. It is reported that 105 pesticides could be listed in the endocrine-disrupting chemical (EDC) group (**Table 1**) [6–54]. Among these 105 pesticides, 31% are fungicides, 21% herbicides, and 46% insecticides; some of these were withdrawn from use several years ago; even a little still can be detected in the environment such as dichloro-diphenyl-trichloroethane (DDT) and atrazine in some countries.

EDCs focused on interfering with endogenous hormones possible by binding to and activating various hormone receptors including estrogen, androgen, thyroid receptors, and aromatase enzymes and mimic the hormone or enzyme activities including agonistic and antagonistic actions. Basically, EDA is mainly related to the reproductive and developmental toxicity. Also the major endocrine pathways would be hypothalamus-pituitary-gonadal and hypothalamus-pituitary-thyroid, and the involving hormones are estrogen, androgen, and thyroid. The Organization for Co-operation and Development (OECD) test guidelines for reproductive and developmental toxicity and EDA are listed in **Table 2** [55, 56]. United States Environmental Protection Agency (US EPA) test guidelines for reproductive and developmental toxicity and EDA are as follows. Guidelines are 870.3550 reproduction/development toxicity screening test, 870.3650 combined repeated dose toxicity with the reproduction/development toxicity screening test, 870.3700 prenatal developmental toxicity study, 870.3800 reproduction and fertility effects, and 870.6300 developmental neurotoxicity study. USEPA Series 890 endocrine disruptor screening program test guidelines are isolated from OPPTS 870 Series. The final endocrine disruptor screening program test guidelines are generally intended to meet testing requirements under Toxic Substances Control Act (TSCA); Federal Insecticide, Fungicide, and Rodenticide Act (FIFRA); and Federal Food, Drug, and Cosmetic Act (FFDCA) to determine if a chemical substance may pose a risk to human health or the environment due to the disruption of the endocrine system. Group A—EDSP Tier 1 and Group B—EDSP Tier 2 test guidelines are listed in **Table 3**.

The main shortcomings of above guidelines are that they are expensive and time-consuming and the need of a lot of number of laboratory animals. It is reported that cost and the minimum number of laboratory animals are requested for applying OECD test guidelines to test toxicity to reproductive and developmental toxicity. **Table 2** shows the cost and minimum number of laboratory animals [55, 56]. Besides, the associated bioethical and social concerns are becoming a challenge. Nowadays, the common knowledge of using laboratory animals is reduce, refine, and replace (3Rs). Facing these situations, we should take cheap and reliable alternatives to screen the reproductive and developmental toxicity and EDA and decide the next steps for necessities of toxicity tests.

It is reported that a widely used technique for screening prenatal developmental toxicity is by monitoring organogenesis during gestational days (GD) 10–12 [57]. In support to whole rat embryo culture (rat WEC), a variety of morphological endpoints is integrated in the total morphological score (TMS) [58]. When applying the TMS in rat WEC, effects of pesticides on

Pesticides	EDC related	Pesticides	EDC related
2,4-D (H)	AR [6]	Heptachlor (I)	ER, AR [25, 46]
Acephate (I)	Hypothalamus [7]	Hexaconazole (F)	Aromatase activity, estrogens, androgens [20]
Acetochlor (H)	ER, TR [8, 9]	Isoproturon (H)	Pregnane X cellular receptor [5]
Alachlor (H)	ER, PR [10, 11]	Iprodione (F)	Aromatase activity, estrogen [2]
Aldicarb (I)	17 Beta-estradiol, progesterone [10, 12]	Linuron (H)	AR, TR [25, 47]
Aldrin (I)	AR [13]	Malathion (I)	TR [10, 48]
Atrazine (H)	Androgen, aromatase activity, estrogen, luteinizing hormone, prolactin [10, 14–17]	Methiocarb (H)	Androgen, estrogen [2]
Bendiocarb (I)	Estrogen effect [10]	Methomyl (I)	Aromatase activity, estrogen [2, 10]
Benomyl (F)	Estrogen, aromatase activity [18]	Methoxychlor (I)	Estrogenic effect, AR, pregnane X cellular receptor [10, 11, 13]
Bioallethrin (I)	Estrogen-sensitive [19]	Metolachlor	Pregnane X cellular receptor [5]
Bitertanol (F)	Aromatase activity, estrogens, androgen [20]	Metribuzin (H)	Hyperthyroidism, somatotropin [49]
Bupirimate (F)	Pregnane X cellular receptor [5]	Mirex (I)	Estrogen effect [10]
Captan (F)	Estrogen action [21]	Molinate (H)	Reduction of fertility [10]
Carbaryl (I)	Estrogen effect [10]	Myclobutanil (F)	Estrogen, androgen, ER, AR, aromatase [20, 21, 35]
Carbendazim (F)	Estrogen and aromatase activity [18]	Nitrofen (H)	Estrogen, androgen [21]
Carbofuran (I)	Progesterone, cortisol, estradiol, testosterone [22]	Oxamyl (I)	Estrogen effect [10]
Chlorothalonil (F)	Androgen-sensitive [23]	Parathion (I)	Melatonin, gonadotrophic hormone [10]
Chlordane (I)	ER [10], AR [13]	Penconazole (F)	Estrogenic effect, aromatase activity, estrogens, androgens [20, 35]
Chlordecone (I)	AE, ER [21, 24, 25]	Pentachlorophenol (H, F, I)	Estrogenic, androgenic affect [10]
Chlorfenvinphos (I)	Estrogen effect [26]	Permethrin (I)	Estrogen-sensitive [19, 29]
Chlorpyrifos methyl (I)	AR [27]	Phenylphenol (F)	Estrogen [50]
Cypermethrin (I)	Estrogenic effect [28, 29]	Prochloraz (F)	Pregnane X cellular receptor, AR, ER, AhR, aromatase activity [2, 5, 36, 51]
Cyproconazole (F)	Aromatase activity, estrogens, androgens [20]	Procymidone (F)	AR [25]
DDT and metabolites (I)	AR, androgen-sensitive, ER, PR [13, 23, 24, 30]	Propamocarb (F)	Aromatase activity, estrogen [2]
Deltamethrin (I)	Estrogenic activity [2]	Propanil (H)	Estrogen [52]

Pesticides	EDC related	Pesticides	EDC related
Diazinon (I)	Estrogenic effect [31]	Propazine (H)	Aromatase activity, estrogen [15]
Dichlorvos (I)	AR [2]	Propiconazole (F)	Estrogen, aromatase activity, androgens [20, 35]
Dicofol (I)	Androgen synthesis, estrogens synthesis, ER [17, 21]	Propoxur (I)	Estrogenic effect [10]
Dieldrin (I)	AR, estrogenic effect, ER [2, 13, 24, 32]	Prothiophos (I)	Estrogenic effect [31]
Diflubenzuron (I)	Pregnane X cellular receptor [5]	Pyridate (H)	ER, AR [21]
Dimethoate (I)	Thyroid hormones, insulin, luteinizing hormone [33, 34]	Pyrifenox (F)	Estrogen [35]
Diuron (H)	Androgen action [17]	Pyriproxyfen (I)	Estrogenic effect [31]
Endosulfan (I)	AR, estrogenic effect, ER, aromatase activity [2, 13, 30, 32]	Resmethrin (I)	Sex hormone [40]
Endrin (I)	AR [13]	Simazine (H)	Aromatase activity, estrogen [15]
Epoxiconazole (F)	Aromatase activity, estrogen, androgens [20, 35]	Sumithrin (I)	Estrogen-sensitive, progesterone [19, 39]
Fenarimol (F)	Androgenic action, aromatase, pregnane X cellular receptor [2, 5, 36]	Tebuconazole (F)	Aromatase activity, estrogens, androgens [20]
Fenbuconazole (F)	Thyroid hormones, pregnane X cellular receptor [5, 10]	Tetramethrin (I)	Estrogen [53]
Fenitrothion (I)	AR, estrogens [21, 37]	Tolclofos-methyl (I)	ER [36]
Fenoxycarb (I)	Testosterone [38]	Toxaphene (I)	Estrogen-sensitive, corticosterone [10, 32]
Fenvalerate (I)	Estrogen-sensitive, progesterone [18, 39]	Triadimefon (F)	Estrogenic effect, aromatase activity, androgens [21]
Fluvalinate (I)	Human sex hormone, progesterone [40, 41]	Triadimenol (F)	Estrogenic effect, aromatase activity, androgens [20, 21]
Flusilazole (F)	Aromatase activity, estrogens, androgens [20]	Tribenuron-methyl (H)	Estrogenic effect [2]
Flutriafol (F)	Estrogen [35]	Trichlorfon (I)	Thyroid function [54]
Glyphosate (H)	Aromatase activity, estrogens [42]	Trifluralin (H)	Pregnane X cellular receptor, steroid hormone [11]
HCB (F)	Thyroid hormone, androgen [43, 44]	Vinclozolin (F)	AR, pregnane X cellular receptor, steroid hormone [2, 11, 25]
HCH (lindane) (I)	Estrous cycles, luteal progesterone, insulin, estradiol, thyroxine, AR, ER, PR [33, 45]		

I, insecticides; F, fungicides; H, herbicides

Table 1. The summary of reported endocrine disruptor pesticides and their related EDC activity.

the embryonic toxicity could be investigated with qualitative and quantitative endpoints. As we know, azoles are antifungal agents for clinical and agricultural use. Penconazole, propiconazole, and triadimefon were most common triazole pesticides in Taiwan. A report

OECD guideline	Topic	Animals	Estimated cost (€)
414	Prenatal development toxicity	784	63,100 (rats) 92,500 (rabbits)
416	Reproductive toxicity in two generations	3200[a]	328,00
421	Screening test for reproductive and developmental toxicity	560	54,600
422	Combined repeated dose toxicity study with the reproduction/developmental toxicity screening test	412	92,000
426	Neurodevelopmental toxicity study	1400	1100

Data came from Rovida and Hartung [55]; Sogorb et al. [56].
[a]All the animals including discarded pups.

Table 2. Economical cost and number of animals needed to apply the OECD guidelines for testing reproductive toxicology.

OPPTS 890 series	Topic
Group A—EDSP Tier 1	
890.1100	Amphibian metamorphosis (frog)
890.1150	Androgen receptor binding (rat prostate)
890.1200	Aromatase (human recombinant)
890.1250	Estrogen receptor binding
890.1300	Estrogen receptor transcriptional activation (human cell line HeLa-9903)
890.1350	Fish short-term reproduction
890.1400	Hershberger (rat)
890.1450	Female pubertal (rat)
890.1500	Male pubertal (rat)
890.1550	Steroidogenesis (human cell line—H295R)
890.1600	Uterotrophic (rat)
Group B—EDSP Tier 2	
890.2100	Avian two-generation toxicity test in the Japanese quail
890.2200	Medaka-extended one-generation reproduction test
890.2300	Larval amphibian growth and development assay (LAGDA)

Table 3. USEPA Tier 1 and Tier 2 test guidelines.

showed that triazole chemicals antagonized the aromatase, which transfer testosterone into 17ß-estradiol in mammals. Triazole chemicals were designed to disrupt the Cyp51 enzyme, which catalyzes the conversion of lanosterol to ergosterol on the fungal cell membrane, and led to cell death when attacked [59]. Though in the respect of mammalian systems Cyp51 is less sensitive to azoles, it was still critical for the sterol biosynthesis pathway and might be related to the thyroid function. In this study, we will take triazoles penconazole, propiconazole, and triadimefon as an example for the alternative of endocrine-disruptor screening.

2. Materials and methods

2.1. Animals

The animal use protocol was reviewed and approved by the Institutional Animal Care and Use Committee of the Taiwan Agricultural Chemicals and Toxic Substances Research Institute. Five-week-old male and female Wistar rats were purchased from BioLASCO (Taipei, Taiwan, ROC). The rats were acclimated to the laboratory environment and reared under a controlled temperature (21 ± 2°C), humidity (40–70%), frequency of ventilation (at least 10/h), and alternating 12 hour cycles of light and darkness. The rats were administered a pellet rodent diet and water ad libitum until they were sacrificed. At 12 weeks of age, the 4 male and 20 female rats were allowed to mate with 2 males to 2 females per day. Gestation day (GD) 0 was defined as the day that sperm was observed in the vagina of the female following mating.

2.2. Chemicals

Materials were obtained from the following manufacturers: DMSO (dimethyl sulfoxide), T3 (triiodothyroxine), Tria (triadimefon), Penc (penconazole), and Prop (propiconazole). All these chemicals with 97% pure at least were purchased from Sigma Chemical Co. (St. Louis, MO).

2.3. Rat whole embryo culture

Five-week-old female and male rats were purchased and reared in the first animal house breeding room until 11–12 weeks of age. Two males and two females were bred in the same cage. The female rats were examined for vaginal plugs on the next day. The occurrence was considered as successful breeding. From the date of pregnancy to the 10.5th day, the embryos were dissected. Reichert's membrane was removed according to the method described by Andrews et al. [60] and Dimopoulou et al. [61], and the embryos containing the intact yolk sac placenta and the urinary membrane were removed and randomly placed in a 4 mL culture medium HBSS solution containing 50 IU of penicillin G/mL and 50 μg streptomycin/mL. The sample was added to a 25 T culture flask containing filter-sterilized rat serum and subjected to complement deactivation and cultured in a constant temperature incubator at 37°C for 48 hours. The culture solution was initially inflated with a mixed gas of 5% O_2, 5% CO_2, and 90% N_2 for 1 minute, and after about 16 hours of culture, 10% O_2, 5% CO_2, and 85% N_2, inflated for 1 minute, and were cultured until the 24th hour. Inflate for 1 minute with 20% O_2, 5% CO_2, and 75% N_2. Each treatment dose was inflated for 1 minute at 40% O_2, 5% CO_2, and 55% N_2 at 40 hours, and the embryos were measured for growth, development, and morphology at the end of 48 hours of culture. Embryonic development was modified according to Brown and Fabro [62], and the evaluation included embryo growth traits and developmental stages, which were considered death if the embryonic yolk sac circulation system or the heart stopped beating. Finally, the carcass head-tail length, developmental grade, head length, number of body segments, and yolk sac diameter were analyzed by t-test and related measurements according to statistical methods; death and abnormal embryos were determined by chi-square. Half of the evaluated embryos were preserved in neutral formalin solution for immunostaining, and the other half were stored in PBS for WB analysis to detect antibody responses related to hormone receptor or enzyme antibodies including AR, ERα, ERß, TRα, TRß, and aromatase.

2.4. Pesticide treatment and evaluation of embryo morphology

This study aimed to investigate the effect of these three pesticides on estrogen receptor (ERα and ERß), thyroid receptor (TRα and TRß), and aromatase activities in whole rat embryo culture (rat WEC) on gestation day (GD) 10.5. The concentrations of WEC were 3.1E-5, 6.2E-5, and 1.2E-4 M of penconazole, propiconazole, and triadimefon. The culture period was 48 hours. After culture the embryo morphology was assessed according to the TMS system [62], we graded the endpoint as no effect (−), little effect (±), effect (+), and potential effect (++). After evaluation of embryo development, it was fixed in formalin or kept in HBSS for immunohistochemistry (IHC) and western blot (WB), respectively.

2.5. Immunohistochemical (IHC) evaluation

The embryos were treated by penconazole, propiconazole, and triadimefon with concentrations of 3.1E-5, 6.2E-5, and 1.2E-4 M. Embryos from control and pesticide treatments were fixed in 10% neutral buffered formalin for 1 week. The embryos were then dehydrated with increasing concentrations of ethanol, cleared in toluene, and embedded in paraffin. All the sections were cut into 5 mm slices and deparaffinized, hydrated, and treated with 0.3% H_2O_2 in PBS (pH 7.6) for 30 minutes to block endogenous peroxidase activity and finally treated with a protein-blocking solution (5% goat serum diluted in phosphate-buffered saline). All these steps were followed by heating the sections in a microwave oven for antigen retrieval using a 0.01 M citrate buffer solution (pH 5.5). Tissue sections were immunostained with rabbit anti-AR(N-20), anti-ER (MC) antibody (Santa Cruz Co., CA), TRα (C0345), TRß (C0346) (Assay Biotechnology Co. Sunnyvale, CA), and aromatase (SM2222P)(Acris Antibodies, Inc., San Diego, CA), which was diluted 1:250 in phosphate-buffered saline and 0.25% bovine serum albumin and maintained at room temperature overnight. The tissue sections were then developed with a streptavidin-HRP kit (Chemicon IHC Select® CA, USA), using diaminobenzidine as the chromogen, and were counterstained with hematoxylin. All images were optimized by using an inverted microscope (Leica, Wetzlar GmbH, Germany). To quantify the relative amount of activity of ER, TR, and aromatase in the IHC, 200 nuclei stained per field in a slide, 5 fields per slide, and 5 slides per dose were counted. The intensity of AR, ER, TR, and aromatase proteins stained in nucleus was graded as (0, negative), + (1, mild), ++ (2, moderate), +++ (3, intense), ++++ (4, more intense), or +++++ (5, very intense). The measurements were control group adjusted, and the values were statistically analyzed.

2.6. Western blot

The embryo homogenates were then centrifuged at 3000 × g for 30 minutes at 4°C. The supernatants were aliquoted and stored at −86°C before use. Before western blotting, protein contents were measured by BCA protein assay (Cat. No. 23225, Pierce). Equal amounts of protein were loaded onto each polyacrylamide gel. The antibody dilutions were 1:200 for the anti-AR (N-20), ERα (MC-20), ERß (H-150) (Santa Cruz Co., CA), TRα (C0345), TRß (C0346) (Assay Biotechnology Co. Sunnyvale, CA), and aromatase (SM2222P) (Acris Antibodies, Inc., San Diego, CA) and 1:5000 for the horseradish peroxidase-conjugated goat anti-rabbit IgG (AP132P, Chemicon International). For each treatment group, five samples were analyzed in two separate blots. Total protein extracts from the embryo homogenates were denatured and separated by sodium dodecyl sulfate-polyacrylamide gel electrophoresis (SDS-PAGE) with 7.5% polyacrylamide. The proteins were transferred to nitrocellulose membranes. The membranes were then blocked for non-specific binding and incubated with polyclonal primary antibodies for AR (N-20), ERα (MC-20), ERß (H-150) (Santa Cruz Co., CA), TRα (C0345), TRß (C0346) (Assay Biotechnology Co. Sunnyvale, CA), aromatase (SM2222P) (Acris Antibodies, Inc., San Diego, CA), and ß-actin (AP132P, Chemicon International). After incubation with primary antibody, the membranes were incubated with horseradish peroxidase-linked anti-goat IgG secondary antibody and visualized on film exposed to enhanced chemiluminescence (VisualizerTM Western Blot Detection Kit, Millipore, MA, USA). The relative amount of protein in the resulting immunoblot bands was estimated by measuring the optical densities of the bands on exposed films using a FOTO/Analyst® Investigator System (Fotodyne Incorporated, WI, USA). The measurements were background adjusted, and the values were statistically analyzed. Protein for ß-actin served as an internal standard.

2.7. Statistical analysis

The values of ER, TR, and aromatase in western blot were normalized against ß-actin. All results were statistically analyzed with the t-test, and $p < 0.05$ was considered statistically significant. The other data were expressed as mean ± SE. Data were subjected to ANOVA followed by *t-test*. The level of significance was set at $p < 0.05$.

3. Results

In the development of rat embryo, 17ß-estradiol (E_2), triiodothyronine (T_3), triadimefon, penconazole, and propiconazole exhibited no significant effect on yolk sac circulatory system, allantois, flexion, heart caudal neural tube, hindbrain, midbrain, forebrain, otic system, optic system, olfactory system, maxillary process, forelimb, hind limb, yolk sac diameter, crown-rump length, head length, and developmental score (**Tables 4–6**; **Figure 1**).

http://dx.doi.org/10.5772/intechopen.81030

Treatment	Yolk sac circulatory system	Allantois	Flexion	Heart	Caudal neural tube	Hindbrain	Midbrain
DMSO	3.1 ± 0.3	4.0 ± 0.0	2.0 ± 0.8	2.6 ± 0.7	3.7 ± 1.3	2.8 ± 0.8	2.8 ± 0.8
E2	3.0 ± 0.8	4.0 ± 0.0	3.0 ± 1.8	2.8 ± 0.5	4.3 ± 1.0	2.0 ± 1.2	2.5 ± 1.0
T3	3.0 ± 0.0	4.0 ± 0.0	2.5 ± 2.1	2.0 ± 1.4	3.0 ± 0.0	3.0 ± 0.0	3.0 ± 0.0
Triadimefon							
L	2.5 ± 0.6	4.0 ± 0.0	3.0 ± 0.8	3.0 ± 0.0	4.0 ± 0.0	1.0 ± 0.0	3.0 ± 0.0
M	2.8 ± 0.5	4.0 ± 0.0	2.5 ± 0.6	3.0 ± 0.0	4.3 ± 0.5	2.5 ± 1.0	2.5 ± 1.0
H	3.0 ± 0.0	4.0 ± 0.0	1.8 ± 1.0	2.8 ± 0.4	4.0 ± 0.9	2.7 ± 0.8	2.7 ± 1.0
Penconazole							
L	3.7 ± 0.6*	4.0 ± 0.0	3.7 ± 1.2*	3.0 ± 0.0	4.3 ± 1.2	3.0 ± 0.0	3.0 ± 0.0
M	3.6 ± 0.6*	4.0 ± 0.0	2.7 ± 0.6	3.0 ± 0.0	4.0 ± 0.0	3.0 ± 0.0	3.0 ± 0.0
H	3.4 ± 0.5	4.0 ± 0.0	3.0 ± 1.9	2.4 ± 0.9	3.8 ± 0.8	2.2 ± 1.1	2.4 ± 0.9
Propiconazole							
L	3.0 ± 0.0	4.0 ± 0.0	3.0 ± 2.0	3.0 ± 0.0	3.7 ± 0.6	2.3 ± 1.2	2.3 ± 1.2
M	2.8 ± 0.4	3.8 ± 0.4	2.4 ± 0.9	3.0 ± 0.0	4.0 ± 0.7	2.8 ± 0.4	2.8 ± 0.5
H	3.0 ± 0.8	4.0 ± 0.0	2.5 ± 1.7	3.0 ± 0.0	3.8 ± 1.0	3.0 ± 0.0	3.0 ± 0.0

All pesticide concentrate are 3.1E-5 M (low concentration, L), 6.2E-5 M (middle concentration, M), and 1.2E-4 M (high concentration, H). Dimethyl sulfoxide, DMSO; 17ß-estradiol, E2; and triiodothyronine, T3. E2 and T3 concentrations, 1.2E-4 M.
*$P < 0.05$.

Table 4. Effect of treatment with triazole pesticides on some developmental scores of rat embryo culture of day 10.5 for 48 hours.

In the immunohistochemistry (IHC), the 17ß-estradiol (ERα and ERß) positive control showed the respective results of receptor expressions. Our results showed that penconazole, propiconazole, and triadimefon induced expressions of ERα (**Figure 2**) and ERß (**Figure 3**) in WEC. This result basically meets the mechanisms of triazoles designed to disrupt the synthesis of steroid hormone. Also, results showed that penconazole, propiconazole, and triadimefon induced expressions of TRß (data not shown), but not in TRα (data not shown) with WEC. The relationship among TRß and AR and ER still needs to be investigated. Also, we need to study the antagonistic effects by adding the antagonists for the receptor expression. These three pesticides did not affect significantly AR (data not shown) and aromatase activity (data not shown). In the western blot (WB) data, these three pesticides did not affect significantly AR, ERα, ERß, TRα, TRß, and aromatase expressions in WEC (data not shown). The difference between IHC and WB induced by these three pesticides might be the sensitivity of detecting method. WB needs some embryos for the protein quantitative, while IHC can detect activity in an embryo.

Treatment	Forebrain	Otic system	Optic system	Olfactory system	Branchial bars	Maxillary process	Mandibular process
DMSO	2.7 ± 0.7	1.8 ± 0.4	2.8 ± 1.3	1.5 ± 0.7	1.4 ± 0.5	0.9 ± 0.3	2.0 ± 0.0
E2	2.8 ± 1.3	2.0 ± 0.8	3.0 ± 1.4	1.0 ± 0.0	1.0 ± 0.0	1.0 ± 0.0	2.0 ± 0.0
T3	3.0 ± 0.0	1.5 ± 0.7	2.5 ± 2.1	1.5 ± 0.7	1.5 ± 0.7	1.0 ± 0.0	2.0 ± 0.0
Triadimefon							
L	2.8 ± 0.6	1.5 ± 0.6	3.5 ± 1.0	1.8 ± 0.5	1.3 ± 0.5	1.0 ± 0.0	2.0 ± 0.0
M	2.3 ± 1.0	1.5 ± 0.6	3.3 ± 1.0	1.0 ± 0.0	1.5 ± 0.6	1.0 ± 0.0	2.0 ± 0.0
H	2.7 ± 1.0	1.7 ± 0.5	3.3 ± 0.8	1.5 ± 0.5	1.2 ± 0.4	1.0 ± 0.0	2.0 ± 0.0
Penconazole							
L	3.3 ± 0.6	1.7 ± 0.6	3.3 ± 1.2	1.7 ± 0.6	1.3 ± 0.6	1.0 ± 0.0	2.0 ± 0.0
M	3.7 ± 0.6	1.7 ± 0.6	4.0 ± 0.0	1.7 ± 0.6	1.7 ± 0.6	1.0 ± 0.0	2.0 ± 0.0
H	2.6 ± 1.5	2.0 ± 1.0	3.2 ± 1.8	1.2 ± 0.8	1.2 ± 0.4	1.0 ± 0.0	2.0 ± 0.0
Propiconazole							
L	2.7 ± 1.5	1.7 ± 1.2	3.3 ± 2.1	1.3 ± 0.6	1.3 ± 0.6	1.0 ± 0.0	2.0 ± 0.0
M	2.8 ± 0.4	1.4 ± 0.5	2.6 ± 1.1	1.2 ± 0.4	1.2 ± 0.4	1.0 ± 0.0	2.0 ± 0.0
H	3.3 ± 0.5	1.5 ± 0.6	2.5 ± 1.7	1.8 ± 0.5	1.0 ± 0.0	1.0 ± 0.0	2.0 ± 0.0

All pesticide concentrate are 3.1E-5 M (low concentration, L), 6.2E-5 M (middle concentration, M), and 1.2E-4 M (high concentration, H). Dimethyl sulfoxide, DMSO; 17ß-estradiol, E2; and triiodothyronine, T3. E2 and T3 concentrations: 1.2E-4 M.

Table 5. Effect of treatment with triazole pesticides on some other developmental scores of rat embryo culture of day 10.5 for 48 hours.

Treatment	Forelimb	Hind limb	Yolk sac diameter (A) (mm)	Yolk sac diameter (B) (mm)	Crown-rump length (mm)	Head length (mm)	Developmental score
DMSO	0.7 ± 0.5	0.7 ± 0.5	6.4 ± 1.2	5.7 ± 1.0	5.2 ± 1.1	1.9 ± 0.6	38 ± 7
E2	0.8 ± 0.5	0.8 ± 0.5	6.6 ± 1.4	5.2 ± 1.7	4.4 ± 1.4	2.2 ± 0.7	38 ± 8
T3	1.0 ± 0.0	1.0 ± 0.0	5.8 ± 0.1	4.9 ± 1.6	4.0 ± 1.8	1.7 ± 0.8	38 ± 6
Triadimefon							
L	0.5 ± 0.6	0.8 ± 0.5	4.8 ± 1.0	4.8 ± 0.6	4.9 ± 0.4	1.7 ± 0.3	40 ± 3
M	0.5 ± 0.6	1.0 ± 0.0	5.0 ± 0.7	5.0 ± 0.7	5.4 ± 1.0	1.9 ± 0.3	38 ± 2
H	0.7 ± 0.5	0.8 ± 0.4	4.7 ± 0.9*	5.3 ± 1.2	4.9 ± 0.9	1.8 ± 0.5	39 ± 4
Penconazole							
L	0.7 ± 0.6	1.3 ± 0.6	7.1 ± 1.7	6.4 ± 1.6	6.0 ± 1.0	2.5 ± 0.6	43 ± 4
M	1.0 ± 0.0	0.7 ± 0.6	6.9 ± 0.5	5.7 ± 1.1	5.8 ± 0.7	3.0 ± 0.5	43 ± 3
H	0.6 ± 0.5	1.0 ± 0.7	6.3 ± 1.2	6.2 ± 1.2	4.6 ± 1.7	2.1 ± 1.1	39 ± 9

Treatment	Forelimb	Hind limb	Yolk sac diameter (A) (mm)	Yolk sac diameter (B) (mm)	Crown-rump length (mm)	Head length (mm)	Developmental score
Propiconazole							
L	0.7 ± 0.6	0.7 ± 0.6	6.0 ± 1.4	5.4 ± 0.8	5.0 ± 0.4	2.1 ± 0.7	38 ± 9
M	0.6 ± 0.5	0.6 ± 0.5	4.2 ± 0.8*	4.5 ± 1.0*	4.5 ± 1.1	1.8 ± 0.4	40 ± 5
H	0.7 ± 0.6	0.8 ± 0.5	5.5 ± 2.2	4.8 ± 0.5	4.2 ± 1.4	1.9 ± 0.8	38 ± 6

All pesticide concentrate are 3.1E-5 M (low concentration, L), 6.2E-5 M (middle concentration, M), and 1.2E-4 M (high concentration, H). Dimethyl sulfoxide, DMSO; 17ß-estradiol, E2; and triiodothyronine, T3. E2 and T3 concentrations: 1.2E-4 M.

*$P < 0.05$.

Table 6. Effect of co-treatment with triazole pesticides on developmental parameters and scores of rat embryo culture of day 10.5 for 48 hours.

4. Discussion

WEC was used to study the prenatal developmental toxicity induced by environmental chemicals including phthalate and methoxyacetic acid [63, 64], aliphatic amides [65], and triazole pesticides [66, 67]. In respect of the 3Rs principle of animal study, WEC is an alternative to screen the potential of prenatal developmental toxicity of environmental compounds. Although ex vivo exposure of WEC was used limitedly without metabolisms of chemicals, most chemicals exhibited their action by parent compound. In this study, we found that in combination with IHC and WB, WEC will be a robust way to detect the endocrine-disrupting activity induced by environmental chemicals. In this study, we used WEC to detect the important receptors including AR, ERα, ERß, TRα, and TRß and enzyme aromatase activity potential induced by triadimefon, penconazole, and propiconazole. There is one shortcoming of WEC to be addressed. Due to the small amount of embryo, WB is hard to quantify the proteins of hormone receptors. The solution to the problem is to pool the embryo treated by one dose and analyze it. Also, we knew that fortunately nowadays IHC quantification is available. Finally, we concluded that in combination with IHC and WB, WEC will be a robust way to detect EDCs in food.

5. Future work and recommendations

In order to meet the 3Rs including reduction, refine, and replace and precise risk assessment, adverse outcome pathway (AOP) is extensively developed by OECD. By tier screening for EDCs, the molecular initiating event (MIE), key event (KE), key event relationship (KER), and adverse outcome (AO) will be studied. As the guideline stated, the AOP framework made clear the mechanisms from MIE, KE, and KER to AO will meet the criteria of 3Rs of the animal study and provide a quick and precise way to regulatory protection goals and decision-making.

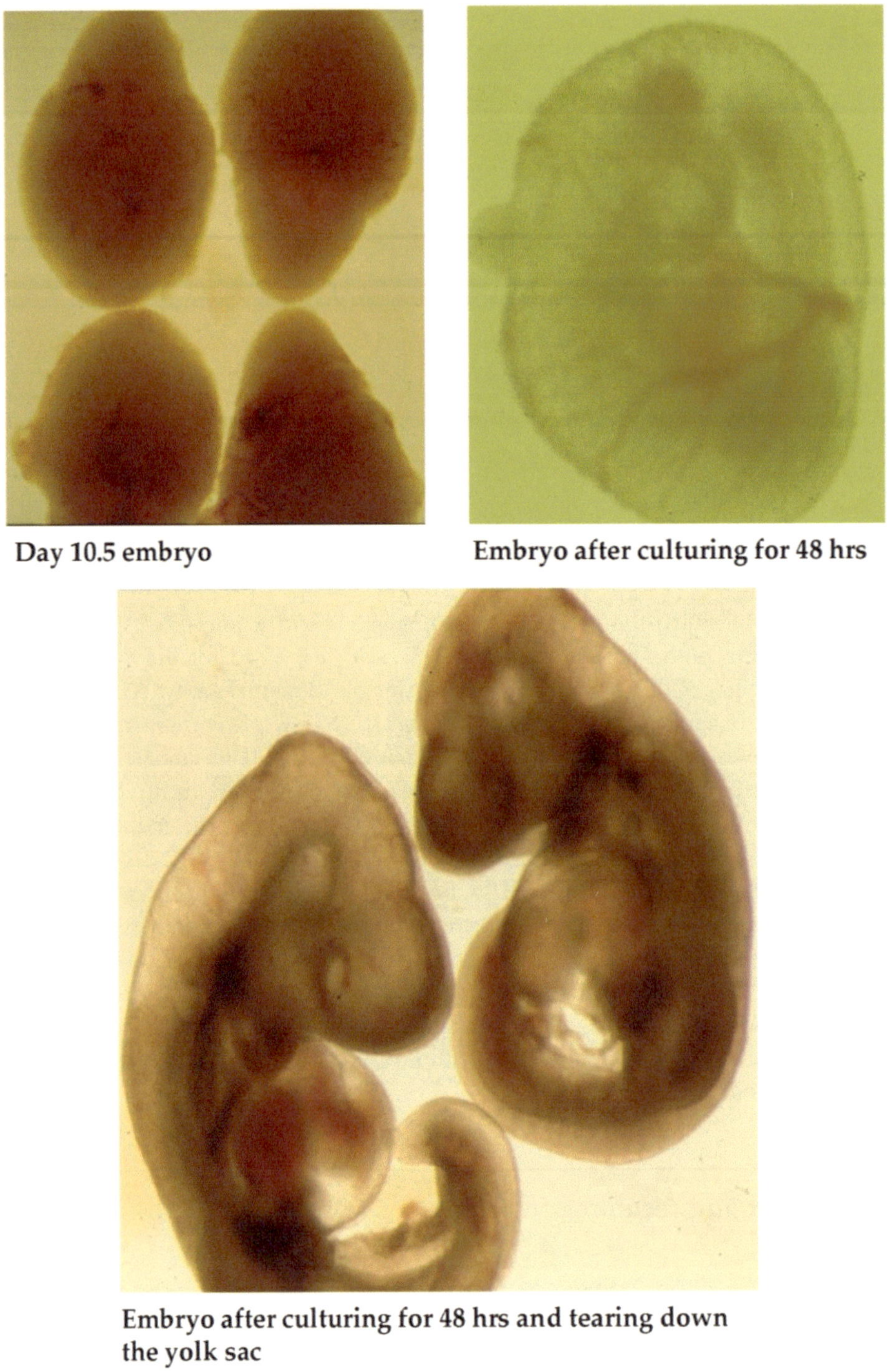

Figure 1. The rat whole embryo culture.

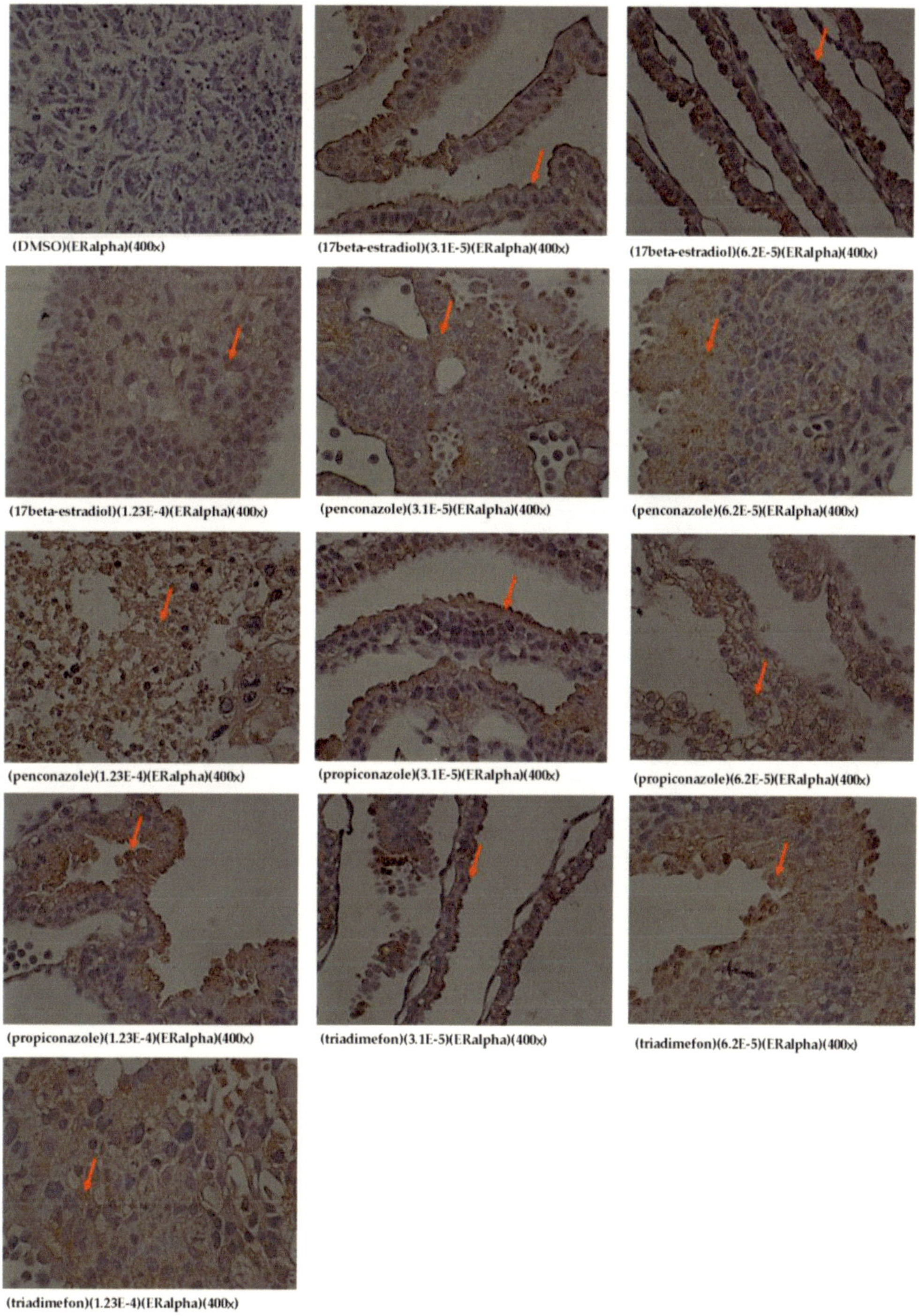

Figure 2. Effect of penconazole, propiconazole, and triadimefon on ERalpha activity in WEC.

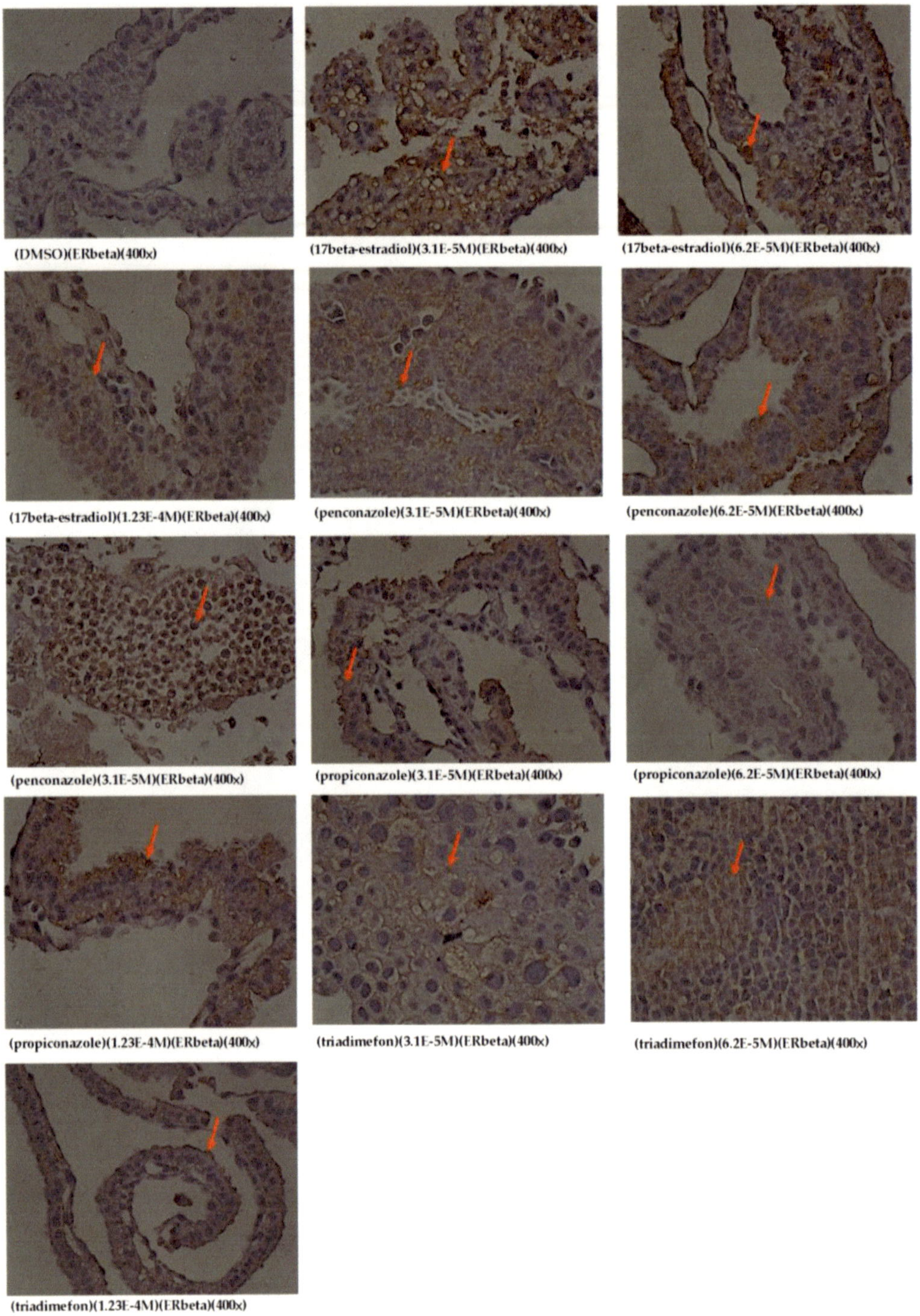

Figure 3. Effect of penconazole, propiconazole, and triadimefon on ERbeta activity in WEC.

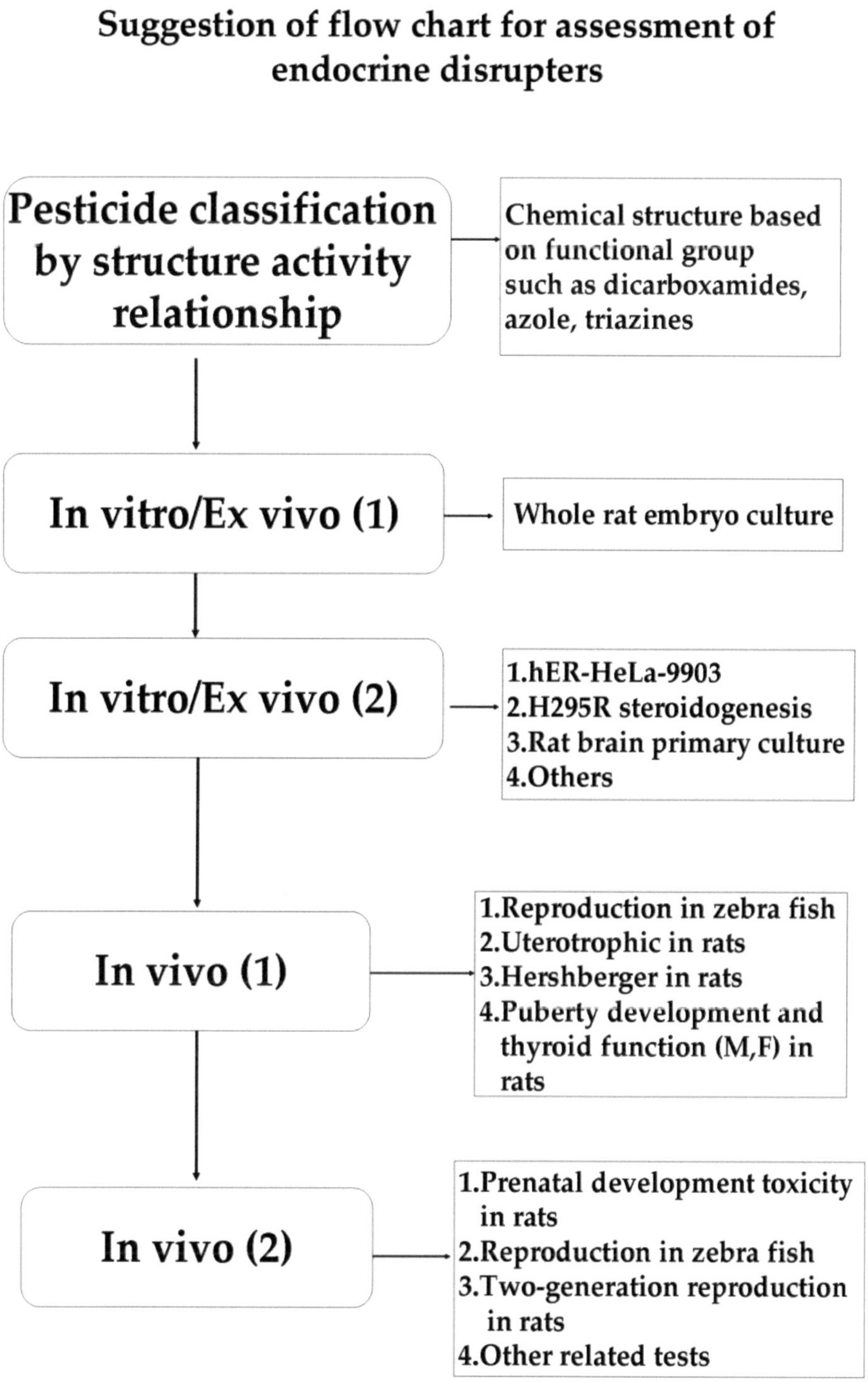

Figure 4. Suggestion of flow chart for assessment of endocrine disrupters.

The overall weight of evidence (WoE) and level of certainty underlying the inference and extrapolation will in turn dictate the most suitable application of the AOP.

6. Diagram/schematic figure

The pragmatic strategy to detect EDA of xenobiotics in food is to take a tier screening. **Figure 4** showed the suggestion of flow chart for assessment of endocrine disruptors. Basically rat embryo culture could be the first screening method except for chemical structure-activity relationship.

7. Conclusions

Penconazole, propiconazole, and triadimefon significantly induced the estrogen receptor expressions. It seems that WEC can be used as a robust method of endocrine-disrupting screening for estrogen receptors.

Acknowledgements

The study was supported partly by the Bureau of Animal and Plant Health Inspection and Quarantine, Council of Agriculture, Executive Yuan, ROC (105AS-10.7.1-PI-P2), and partly by National Health Research Institutes, Zhunan, Miaoli County 35053, ROC (NHRI-106A1-PDCO-3416181).

Conflicts of interest

The authors declare no conflicts of interest.

Abbreviations

MRL	maximum residue level
EDCs	endocrine-disrupting chemicals
OECD	Organization for Economic Co-operation and Development
OPPTS	The Office of Prevention, Pesticides, and Toxic Substances
rat WEC	whole rat embryo culture

AR	androgen receptor
ERα	estrogen receptor alpha
ERß	estrogen receptor beta
TRα	thyroid receptor alpha
TRß	thyroid receptor beta
IHC	immunohistochemistry
WB	western blot

Author details

Shui-Yuan Lu[1]*, Pinpin Lin[2], Wei-Ren Tsai[1] and Chen-Yi Weng[2]

*Address all correspondence to: lusueyen@tactri.gov.tw

1 Applied Toxicology Division, Taiwan Agricultural Chemicals and Toxic Substances Research Institute (TACTRI), Council of Agriculture, Executive Yuan, Taichung, Taiwan, R.O.C.

2 National Institute of Environmental Health Sciences, National Health Research Institutes (NHRI), Miaoli County, Taiwan, R.O.C.

References

[1] Vinggaard AM, Hnida C, Breinholt V, Larsen JC. Screening of selected pesticides for inhibition of CYP19 aromatase activity in vitro. Toxicology In Vitro. 2000;**14**:227-234

[2] Andersen HR, Cook SJ, Waldbillig D. Effects of currently used pesticides in assays for estrogenicity, androgenicity, and aromatase activity in vitro. Toxicology and Applied Pharmacology. 2002;**179**:1-12

[3] Kojima H, Katsura E, Takeuchi S, Niiyama K, Kobayashi K. Screening for estrogen and androgen receptor activities in 200 pesticides by in vitro reporter gene assays using Chinese hamster ovary cells. Environmental Health Perspectives. 2004;**112**:524-531

[4] Lemaire G, Mnif W, Mauvais P, Balaguer P, Rahmani R. Activation of alpha- and beta-estrogen receptors by persistent pesticides in reporter cell lines. Life Sciences. 2006;**79**: 1160-1169

[5] Lemaire G, Mnif W, Pascussi JM, Pillon A, Rabenoelina F, Fenet H, et al. Identification of new human PXR ligands among pesticides using a stable reporter cell system. Toxicological Sciences. 2006;**91**:501-509

[6] Kim DO, Lee SK, Jeon TW, Jin CH, Hyun SH, Kim EJ, et al. Role of metabolism in parathion-induced hepatotoxicity and immunotoxicity. Journal of Toxicology and Environmental Health, Part A. 2005;**68**:2187-2205

[7] Singh AK. Acute effects of acephate and methamidophos and interleukin-1 on corticotropin-releasing factor (CRF) synthesis in and release from the hypothalamus in vitro. Comparative Biochemistry and Physiology, Part C: Toxicology & Pharmacology. 2002;**132**:9-24

[8] Rollerová EE. Interaction of acetochlor with estrogen receptor in the rat uterus. Acetochlor —Possible endocrinemodulator? General Physiology and Biophysics. 2000;**19**:73-84

[9] Crump D, Werry K, Veldhoen N, Van Aggelen G, Helbing CC. Exposure to the herbicide acetochlor alters thyroid hormone-dependent gene expression and metamorphosis in *Xenopus laevis*. Environmental Health Perspectives. 2002;**110**:1199-1205

[10] Cocco P. On the rumors about the silent spring. Review of the scientific evidence linking occupational and environmental pesticide exposure to endocrine disruption health effects. Cadernos de Saúde Pública. 2002;**18**:379-402

[11] Mikamo E, Harada S, Nishikawa J, Nishihara T. Endocrine disruptors induce cytochrome P450 by affecting transcriptional regulation via Pregnane X receptor. Toxicology and Applied Pharmacology. 2003;**193**:66-72

[12] Klotz D, Arnold SF, McLachlan JA. Inhibition of 17 beta-estradiol and progesterone activity in human breast and endometrial cancer cells by carbamate insecticides. Life Sciences. 1997;**60**:1467-1475

[13] Lemaire G, Terouanne B, Mauvais P, Michel S, Rahmani R. Effect of organochlorine pesticides on human androgen receptor activation in vitro. Toxicology and Applied Pharmacology. 2004;**196**:235-246

[14] Cooper R, Stoker TE, Tyrey L, Goldman JM, McElroy WK. Atrazine disrupts the hypothalamic control of pituitary-ovarian function. Toxicological Sciences. 2000;**53**:297-307

[15] Sanderson JT, Seinen W, Giesy JP, van den Berg M. 2-Chloro-s-triazine herbicides induce aromatase (CYP19) activity in H295R human adrenocortical carcinoma cells, a novel mechanism for estrogenicity? Toxicological Sciences. 2000;**54**:121-127

[16] Hayes T, Tsui M, Hoang A, Haeffele C, Vonk A. Atrazine-induced hermaphroditism at 0.1 ppb in American leopard frogs (*Rana pipiens*); laboratory and field evidence. Environmental Health Perspectives. 2003;**111**:568-575

[17] Thibaut R, Porte C. Effects of endocrine disrupters on sex steroid synthesis and metabolism pathways in fish. The Journal of Steroid Biochemistry and Molecular Biology. 2004; **92**:485-494

[18] Morinaga H, Yanase T, Nomura M, Okabe T, Goto K, Harada N, et al. A benzimidazole fungicide; benomyl; and its metabolite; carbendazim; induce aromatase activity in a human ovarian granulose-like tumor cell line (KGN). Endocrinology. 2004;**145**:1860-1869

[19] Kim IY, Shin JH, Kim HS, Lee SJ, Kang IH, Kim TS, et al. Assessing estrogenic activity of pyrethroid insecticides using in vitro combination assays. The Journal of Reproduction and Development. 2004;**50**:245-255

[20] Trosken EE, Scholz K, Lutz RW, Volkel W, Zarn JA, Lutz WK. Comparative assessment of the inhibition of recombinant human CYP19 (aromatase) by azoles used in agriculture and as drugs for humans. Endocrine Research. 2004;**30**:387-394

[21] Okubo T, Yokoyama Y, Kano K, Soya Y, Kano I. Estimation of estrogenic and antiestrogenic activities of selected pesticides by MCF-7 cell proliferation assay. Archives of Environmental Contamination and Toxicology. 2004;**46**:445-453

[22] Goad R, Goad J, Atieh B, Gupta R. Carbofuran-induced endocrine disruption in adult male rats. Toxicology Mechanisms and Methods. 2004;**14**:233-239

[23] Tessier D, Matsumura F. Increased ErbB-2 tyrosine kinase activity; MAPK phosphorylation; and cell proliferation in the prostate cancer cell line LNCaP following treatment by select pesticides. Toxicological Sciences. 2001;**60**:38-43

[24] Tapiero HT, Nguyen BG, Tew KD. Estrogens and environmental estrogens. Biomedicine & Pharmacotherapy. 2002;**56**:36-44

[25] Fang H, Tong W, Branham WS, Moland CL, Dial SL, Hong H, et al. Study of 202 natural; synthetic; and environmental chemicals for binding to the androgen receptor. Chemical Research in Toxicology. 2003;**16**:1338-1358

[26] Vinggaard A, Breinholt V, Larsen JC. Screening of selected pesticides for oestrogen receptor activation in vitro. Food Additives and Contaminants. 1999;**16**:533-542

[27] Kang HG, Jeong SH, Cho JH, Kim DG, Park JM, Cho MH. Chlropyrifos-methyl shows anti-androgenic activity without estrogenic activity in rats. Toxicology. 2004;**199**:219-230

[28] Chen H, Xiao J, Hu G, Zhou J, Xiao H, Wang X. Estrogenicity of organophosphorus and pyrethroid pesticides. Journal of Toxicology and Environmental Health, Part A. 2002;**65**: 1419-1435

[29] McCarthy AR, Thomson BM, Shaw IC, Abella AD. Estrogenicity of pyrethroid insecticide metabolites. Journal of Environmental Monitoring. 2006;**8**:197-202

[30] Bulayeva NN, Watson CS. Xenoestrogen-induced ERK-1 and ERK-2 activation via multiple membrane-initiated signaling pathways. Environmental Health Perspectives. 2004; **112**:1481-1487

[31] Manabe M, Kanda S, Fukunaga K, Tsubura A, Nishiyama T. Evaluation of the estrogenic activities of some pesticides and their combinations using MtT/Se cell proliferation assay. International Journal of Hygiene and Environmental Health. 2006;**209**:413-421

[32] Soto AM, Chung KL, Sonnenschein C. The pesticides endosulfan; toxaphene; and dieldrin have estrogenic effects on human estrogen-sensitive cells. Environmental Health Perspectives. 1994;**102**:380-383

[33] Rawlings NC, Cook SJ, Waldbillig D. Effects of the pesticides carbofuran; chlorpyrifos; dimethoate; lindane; triallate; trifluralin; 2;4-D; and pentachlorophenol on the metabolic endocrine and reproductive endocrine system in ewes. Journal of Toxicology and Environmental Health, Part A. 1998;**54**:21-36

[34] Mahjoubi-Samet A, Hamadi F, Soussia L, Fadhel G, Zeghal N. Dimethoate effects on thyroid function in suckling rats. Annales d'Endocrinologie. 2005;**66**:96-104

[35] Hurst MRR, Sheahan DA. The potential for estrogenic effects of pesticides in headwater streams in the UK. Science of the Total Environment. 2003;**301**:87-96

[36] Grunfeld HT, Bonefeld-Jorgensen EC. Effect of in vitro estrogenic pesticides on human estrogen receptor alpha and beta mRNA levels. Toxicology Letters. 2004;**151**:467-480

[37] Tamura H, Yoshikawa H, Gaido KW, Ross SM, DeLisle RK, Welsh WJ, et al. Interaction of organophosphate pesticides and related compounds with the androgen receptor. Environmental Health Perspectives. 2003;**111**:545-552

[38] Verslycke T. Testosterone and energy metabolism in the estuarine mysid *Neomysis* integer (*Crustacea, Mysidacea*) following exposure to endocrine disruptors. Environmental Toxicology and Chemistry. 2004;**23**:1289-1296

[39] Garey J, Wolff MS. Estrogenic and antiprogestagenic activities of pyrethroid insecticides. Biochemical and Biophysical Research Communications. 1998;**251**:855-859

[40] Eil CC, Nisula BC. The binding properties of pyrethroids to human skin fibroblast androgen receptors and to sex hormone binding globulin. Journal of Steroid Biochemistry. 1990; **35**:409-414

[41] Chen HY, Liu R, He J, Song L, Bian Q, Xu L, et al. Effects of fenvalerate on progesterone production in cultured rat granulosa cells. Reproductive Toxicology. 2005;**20**:195-202

[42] Richard S, Moslemi S, Sipahutar H, Benachour N, Seralini G-E. Differential effects of glyphosate and roundup on human placental cells and aromatase. Environmental Health Perspectives. 2005;**113**:716-720

[43] Ralph JJ, Orgebin-Crist MC, Lareyre JJ, Nelson CC. Disruption of androgen regulation in the prostate by the environmental contaminant hexachlorobenzene. Environmental Health Perspectives. 2003;**111**:461-466

[44] Verreault J, Skaare JU, Jenssen BM, Gabrielsen GW. Effects of organochlorine contaminants on thyroid hormone levels in Arctic breeding glaucous gulls; *Larus hyperboreus*. Environmental Health Perspectives. 2004;**112**:532-537

[45] Beard AB, Rawlings NC. Thyroid function and effects on reproduction in ewes exposed to the organochlorine pesticides lindane or pentachlorophenol (PCP) from conception. Journal of Toxicology and Environmental Health, Part A. 1999;**58**:509-530

[46] Oduma JA, Wango EO, Oduor-Okelo D, Makawiti DW, Odongo H. In vivo and in vitro effects of graded doses of the pesticide heptachlor on female sex steroid production in rats.

Comparative Biochemistry and Physiology, Part C, Pharmacology, Toxicology & Endocrinology. 1995;**111**:191-196

[47] Schmutzler C, Gotthardt I, Hofmann PJ, Radovic B, Kovacs G, Stemmler L, et al. Endocrine disruptors and the thyroid gland—A combined in vitro and in vivo analysis of potential new biomarkers. Environmental Health Perspectives. 2007;**115**:77-83

[48] Ishihara A, Nishiyama N, Sugiyama S, Yamauchi K. The effect of endocrine disrupting chemicals on thyroid hormone binding to Japanese quail transthyretin and thyroid hormone receptor. General and Comparative Endocrinology. 2003;**134**:36-43

[49] Porter W, Green SM, Debbink NL, Carlson I. Groundwater pesticides, interactive effects of low concentrations of carbamates aldicarb and methomyl and the triazine metribuzin on thyroxine and somatotropin levels in white rats. Journal of Toxicology and Environmental Health. 1993;**40**:15-34

[50] Sonnenschein C, Soto AM. An updated review of environmental estrogen and androgen mimics and antagonists. The Journal of Steroid Biochemistry and Molecular Biology. 1998; **65**:143-150

[51] Vinggaard AM, Hass U, Dalgaard M, Andersen HR, Bonefeld-Jørgensen E, Christiansen S, et al. Prochloraz, an imidazole fungicide with multiple mechanisms of action. International Journal of Andrology. 2006;**29**:186-192

[52] Salazar KD, Schafer R, Barnett JB, Miller MR. Evidence for a novel endocrine disruptor, the pesticide propanil requires the ovaries and steroid synthesis to enhance humoral immunity. Toxicological Sciences. 2006;**93**:62-74

[53] Kim SS, Kwack SJ, Lee RD, Lim KJ, Rhee GS, Seok JH, et al. Assessment of estrogenic and androgenic activities of tetramethrin in vitro and in vivo assays. Journal of Toxicology and Environmental Health, Part A. 2005;**68**:2277-2289

[54] Nicolau GG. Circadian rhythms of RNA; DNA and protein in the rat thyroid; adrenal and testis in chronic pesticide exposure. III. Effects of the insecticides (dichlorvos and trichlorphon). Physiologie. 1983;**20**:93-101

[55] Rovida C, Hartung T. Re-evaluation of animal numbers and costs for in vivo tests to accomplish REACH legislation requirements for chemicals: A report by the transatlantic think tank for toxicology (t(4)). ALTEX. 2009;**26**:187-208

[56] Sogorb MA, Pamies D, de Lapuente J, Estevan C, Estúvez J, Vilanova E. An integrated approach for detecting embryotoxicity and developmental toxicity of environmental contaminants using in vitro alternative methods. Toxicology Letters. 2014;**230**:356-367

[57] New DA, Coppola PT, Cockroft DL. Comparison of growth in vitro and in vivo of postimplantation rat embryos. Journal of Embryology and Experimental Morphology. 1976;**36**: 133-144

[58] Piersma AH. Validation of alternative methods for developmental toxicity testing. Toxicology Letters. 2004;**149**:147-153

[59] Marotta F, Tiboni GM. Molecular aspects of azoles-induced teratogenesis. Expert Opinion on Drug Metabolism & Toxicology. 2010;**6**:461-482

[60] Andrews JE, Ebron-McCoy M, Logsdon TR, Mole LM, Kavlock RJ, Rogers JM. Developmental toxicity of methanol in whole embryo culture: A comparative study with mouse and rat embryos. Toxicology. 1993;**81**:205-215

[61] Dimopoulou M, Verhoef A, Pennings JLA, van Ravenzwaay B, Rietjens IMCM, Piersma AH. A transcriptomic approach for evaluating the relative potency and mechanism of action of azoles in the rat whole embryo culture. Toxicology. 2017;**392**:96-105

[62] Brown NA, Fabro S. Quantitation of rat embryonic development in vitro: A morphological scoring system. Teratology. 1981;**24**:65-78

[63] Robinson JF, van Beelen VA, Verhoef A, Renkens MF, Luijten M, van Herwijnen MH, et al. Embryotoxicant-specific transcriptomic responses in rat postimplantation whole-embryo culture. Toxicological Sciences. 2010;**118**:675-685. Erratum in: Toxicological Sciences. 2011; **120**:529

[64] Robinson JF, Verhoef A, van Beelen VA, Pennings JL, Piersma AH. Dose-response analysis of phthalate effects on gene expression in rat whole embryo culture. Toxicology and Applied Pharmacology. 2012;**264**:32-41

[65] Flick B, Talsness CE, Jäckh R, Buesen R, Klug S. Embryotoxic potential of N-methyl-pyrrolidone (NMP) and three of its metabolites using the rat whole embryo culture system. Toxicology and Applied Pharmacology. 2009;**237**:154-167

[66] de Jong E, Barenys M, Hermsen SA, Verhoef A, Ossendorp BC, Bessems JG, et al. Comparison of the mouse embryonic stem cell test, the rat whole embryo culture and the zebrafish embryotoxicity test as alternative methods for developmental toxicity testing of six 1,2,4-triazoles. Toxicology and Applied Pharmacology. 2011;**253**:103-111

[67] Robinson JF, Tonk EC, Verhoef A, Piersma AH. Triazole induced concentration-related gene signatures in rat whole embryo culture. Reproductive Toxicology. 2012;**34**:275-283